It's Not Always Like This, But It Is Now

A Guide to Letting Go of Depression and Simply Living Well

Josh Blumenthal

Playa Publishing
www.PlayaPublishing.com

Note: Information contained in this book is intended as an educational aid only. While every effort has been made to ensure its accuracy, in no way is this book intended to replace, countermand, or conflict with the advice or treatment provided by a medical professional. The author and publisher specifically disclaim any and all liability arising directly or indirectly from the use or application of any information contained in this book. The ultimate decision concerning care should be made between you and your doctor.

ISBN 978-0-9838167-0-6

Printed in the United States of America.

Dedicated to You and Me

Contents

Chapter 1

Why Can't I Just Be Happy?

Think about the beauty of a skyscraper climbing high into the sky. Now imagine that same skyscraper is filled with dynamite. It wouldn't take but a few seconds to destroy the building, sending it crashing to the ground; but it would take years of work to rebuild it. Your life is much the same way. In an instant, so much can be destroyed and taken away; but through the effort you make to rebuild your life, you can make it worthwhile once again.

I took this path from depression to a life of appreciation. I rediscovered the world I had long forgotten and the happiness I thought was gone forever, but there was no single realization that changed my life, no experience that suddenly made me better. It took time, effort, and patience; but I prevailed. And to this day, I must constantly remind myself of the lessons I have learned and the actions I must carry out in order to fend off depression.

You see, for someone who has been through depression, it's easy for it to return if you stop committing the actions you used to overcome it. It's easy to return because the lessons I learned and have included in this book are not just about overcoming depression but about living well. So too, those who have never before known depression may be headed that way if they do not reevaluate their lives and make necessary changes.

This book is not so much about me as it is about life. It's about the journey of getting to know yourself, getting to know the world around you, and developing your relationship with each. The discussions and techniques in this guide are about making the most of what you have, letting go of what you no longer need, and learning to appreciate what's benefiting you—in essence, taking control of your life. The journey you will take, however, is not dependent on this book but on you.

The most important thing you can know throughout the journey you are about to embark on is that no one is going to get you through this but you. Many people will be available throughout your life to help you as I am now, but you are the one who must make the effort. There is a world of acceptance, joy, and gratitude ahead; but this process will not always be easy. However, few things that are worthwhile ever come with ease.

In every moment, you have a choice. The choice you have in this moment is to continue on the path you have been walking or choose a new direction with a new opportunity for happiness. This new direction may come with occasional doubt. This new opportunity may cause you to reconsider beliefs you hold dear. But this new path is where strength, confidence, and happiness reside. This is a journey that begins with your effort and continues the rest of your life. I did it, and believe me, so can you.

Welcome to your life. I promise you it's worth the effort.

Your Journey

The first step in your journey is a simple but important one. It involves making a single commitment to yourself. Before we move ahead, you must make the promise that you won't harm yourself in any way. This means both physically and mentally. Anything you are doing or considering doing that involves harming yourself must be given up. This journey is not about escaping your life; it's about embracing it, and making this promise to yourself is the first step in reaching for that embrace.

Particularly if you have gone so far as to consider or attempt suicide, it's important to understand that what you are truly seeking is not an end to your life but an end to your suffering. Relief, however, is a human emotion that can only be felt while you are still alive, and there is no relief in suicide. The only guarantee I can make you about pain, relief, and the future is that every path you take in life and every decision you make will at some point lead to good fortune except suicide. There are, however, very useful ways to find the relief you seek; but you won't get there if you don't make this commitment.

The reality is that you didn't just pick up this book because you think your life needs improvement; you picked up this book because you believe *you can* improve your life. So if you haven't yet made that promise to yourself, now is the time to do it. "I promise I will not harm myself." Now say it out loud so that you hear the importance of your own words. "I promise I will not harm myself."

Your greatest strength in this journey will be your ability to remain genuine, and that means accepting yourself. Even if you do not like the person you are right now, you will soon learn that accepting things the way they are is what leads to appreciation while rejecting what exists leads to depression. You must, therefore, give up your rejection of yourself by embracing a life in which you uplift yourself. And this is what this first step is all about.

Now that you've taken your first step toward not harming yourself, it's time to make your next step about healing yourself. While the first step involved a promise, this next step involves action. It is equally as simple and equally as valuable: *Go for a walk outside.* Although you may be in a place right now in which leaving the indoors is not an option, the sooner you can get outside, the faster you will begin the healing process. If you're inside and not dressed, get dressed, put on your shoes, grab your keys, and head out the door with this book. You need to get out into the world where there is breathing room and fresh air, and you won't find that indoors.

While you are outside, consider kicking up the speed of that walk into a short run. It doesn't matter how far you run. Simply doing it can make a significant difference in your life as I have witnessed so many people use running to improve their state of mind. This journey does not just involve improving the way you feel emotionally but improving the way you feel physically; however, you will soon discover how connected your emotional and physical health really are.

Going for a walk or run is the first physical step in your journey. By taking this step outdoors, you stop closing yourself off to the world by remaining inside. You must remember that the world extends far beyond the confining walls of the indoors. By walking outside, you begin to reconnect with everything around you, a relationship you may have forgotten about.

What Is Depression?

To me, depression is the realization that you are unsatisfied with your life without the knowledge of how or motivation to do something about it. Depression is expressed in several ways. Sometimes you don't feel. You don't smile and you can't cry. You are indifferent to most everything that comes your way and don't understand why you can't just be happy. Essentially, you are numb. Other times, it is many depressive emotions hitting you at once, causing feelings of loneliness, sadness, anxiety, and defeat. In both cases, you give up on yourself, believing there is no resolution. Nearly everything but you seems to be in motion. You have nothing solid and see no evidence of betterment. Hard times don't help to make you stronger but only make you more exhausted and weak.

Depression often follows the loss of something in which you have invested considerable energy. Maybe it was the loss of a relationship with another person. Maybe it was the loss of your job, health, or way of life. It may have been something that happened a while ago and you didn't realize its impact at the time like giving up on a dream. It may have been an event from your past that bothered you at the time and continues to affect you negatively today like rape, abuse, or someone's death, which translates to the loss of your personal comfort and security. It may even have been something that you don't remember at all. Regardless of what may have led to your depression, it is less important than you may realize because this book is not about finding your personal trigger; it's about letting go of it.

You may have become dissatisfied with your life for any number of reasons, but the way you regularly interact with this world reinforces that feeling. People often encounter the same type of experiences repeatedly in their lives, albeit with different circumstances. For example, some people nearly always feel taken advantage of whereas others nearly always feel appreciative of their encounters in a variety of different situations. This is because circumstances themselves don't determine the course of your life; the way you approach them and react to them determines it.

Like everyone, you have a general set of perspectives about people, relationships, yourself, and many other parts of this world. These perspectives you have guide your actions, which is why seemingly different situations continue to result in similar outcomes. And every day, as you communicate with people, react to situations, and interpret your experiences in habitual ways, you confirm your existing perspectives on life.

Through conceptual discussions and physical techniques, this guide will help you reevaluate and change many of the ways you view your life and interact with this world. Changing the way you are living may at times conflict with what you want to do, but I am not trying to help you do what you want to do; I am trying to help you feel how you want to feel. Every situation you encounter has one thing in common: you—and depending on how you address your circumstances, you determine whether you come away from a situation better or worse off.

Those with depression typically make bad decisions, socialize with the wrong people, and attach to the wrong feelings. They feel lost and avoid focusing on their lives through distractions like television, drugs, the internet, other people, work, and sleep. However, distractions simply allow for the temporary halt of depression rather than confronting the difficult issues of life and making real change. Betterment has to come from the inside-out or the feelings of depression will appear every time there is a lull in external stimulation.

Many, however, believe these distractions are what make their days livable. They may fear that taking action could make their lives worse; they may be unaware of how to make positive change, or they may simply believe that their lives are hopeless. However, it's only when the distractions end and your daily routines come to a halt that you discover how you truly feel.

Rather than compulsively avoiding examining yourself through distraction, experience your emotions. Pretending to be someone else or hiding the way you feel will only make it more difficult to overcome depression. Don't worry if you are unsure of who you are in this moment. If you are open to exploring yourself and learning about this world, you will soon discover who you are and create a life that makes you feel good.

Depression exists in your life as a result of you not living in ways that support a healthy relationship with yourself and the world around you. This is because pain resonates. It draws your attention to help you learn lessons about what you should and shouldn't do as well as signaling the urgent need to focus on healing yourself. Right now, depression may feel like a horrible plague in your life; but it is actually providing you a great gift. Your depression feels painful because it is a warning trying to tell you that your perspectives, actions, and focus aren't working for you; and unless you make positive change, things will only get worse. Lucky for you, you've already taken the first steps in the journey of making positive change.

As you read this book, I encourage you to focus less on eliminating depression and more on bettering your life. If you view overcoming depression as your goal, every time you feel bad, you will believe you are failing. On the other hand, when you view your goal as improving your life, the work is constant. You will not recognize uncomfortable moments as reasons to condemn yourself but opportunities to examine yourself.

Since this book is at its core about improving your life, even those who are *not* diagnosed with clinical depression can gain a great deal from the lessons within. Some discussions may not always apply to you; however, understanding the depths of depression can help you avoid ending up there in the future.

I am not a doctor and, therefore, will not advocate or condemn the use of prescription medicine to help you through your journey. The only comment I will make about antidepressants and anti-anxiety drugs is that while they can offer several benefits, including giving patients breathing room to handle problems and the ability to reason better, they are not a long-term cure for depression.[1] So regardless of whether you choose to take prescription medicine for depression, it is essential that you change your lifestyle, both the way you act and the way you think.

Now there will undoubtedly be those who believe that depression cannot be overcome through a change in behavior because of chemical imbalances in the brain. While there are circumstances in which some people need professional assistance, several chemical imbalances linked to depression *can* be overcome through behavioral changes. In Chapter 2, I will discuss certain chemicals in the brain that affect feelings of pleasure and how you can increase their prevalence in your body through your actions, both in how you interact with the world around you as well as what you put into your body.

Likewise, there are probably those who believe they are too old, unintelligent, or in some way incapable of changing their lives. I can guarantee that if you are willing to use "who you are" as an excuse for not going after or accomplishing what you want, you will never be completely satisfied in your life. Depression leaves a lot of room for improvement. And that "room" is called opportunity.

About the Author

So what makes me an authority figure on the subject of depression if I don't have a degree in psychology? Well, I am just like you. I've been through depression...many times. I've been confused, scared, lonely, numb, and found myself crying without any provoking. I've been to the brink of suicide and had the paramedics arrive at my doorstep. I've made myself physically ill with my thoughts. I've taken medication for depression and read books on the subject. I've been to psychologists, psychiatrists, therapists, and hypnotherapists; and some of them even gave up on me, but I never did.

There was a time when I would wake up every day feeling miserable, criticizing the world, and wishing my life had turned out differently. I had always believed that I deserved happiness, and yet it was nowhere to be found—at least as far as I could see. I spent so long being cynical. Nothing and no one was ever good enough. I thought I was always right. I wouldn't compromise. I judged others and feared others judged me. I walked away from people when I was upset and chased after them when they left me. I made mistakes and mourned my life, constantly thinking how my life would have been better had I made different choices.

That was my life, but today I am no longer that person. I live a new life, a better one. I chose not to close the book on my life but to explore it, and what I found was a world waiting for me to step up and make the most of what existed rather than demanding what I wished existed. The truth is that I do not always have it easy or get everything I want, but I have become proud of who I am. And in overcoming depression, appreciating yourself is more important than anything this world could ever give you.

My course of study was and still is life as I've come to realize what it takes not just to overcome depression but to avoid its return. In the end, it took a conscious effort on my own part to pay attention to what was happening in my life, understand how I was approaching my experiences, and make personal changes to employ the lessons I learned. It was on me to accept things the way they were and put forth effort to improve my life just as you must put forth effort to improve yours.

It is truly an unusual yet relieving feeling after depression when you see promise and beauty in the world, and then all of a sudden, you get bad news and it doesn't seem as terrible as you think it should feel. You realize you have an opportunity to make the most of what happened. And so you do.

Throughout my experiences with depression and subsequent recovery, I documented the journey as I overcame this shadow. I took the time to evaluate my thoughts, feelings, and experiences in an effort to understand why I wasn't happy and what I was doing wrong. I learned lessons about myself and this world, and I made the effort to change the way I approached the two. As I began feeling better, I listened to the stories of friends, family, and colleagues; and I realized I had not been alone in the way I had felt.

I found so many people who were unhappy, unsatisfied, and spending much of their days wondering why life had to be so hard. They felt neglected, disrespected, and that they were often treated unfairly. No matter how hard they tried, they seemed unimpressed with life, waiting for the axe to fall—sometimes wishing for it to fall.

In a world that seemed so unhappy, I wondered why. So I opened myself up to others, discussed their dilemmas with them, shared my thoughts, and recognized familiar tendencies. I discovered that while experiences make us all different people and we each are sensitive to different emotional triggers, there are similar perspectives prevalent among those who are depressed. They are perspectives I too once held and know to be traps of uneasiness.

Some of these perspectives had come from advice that just wasn't very good. Other perspectives had come from valuable advice that was simply misinterpreted. Too much of the time, it seemed for me and for others that we were all misunderstanding the way basic concepts play roles in our lives. It seemed like we would take advice and then essentially walk away from depression only to circle back around to it again.

It was at that point that I knew I had a responsibility to share my breakthroughs with others. In this book, I focus on the universal themes that affect the way we all view and interact with ourselves and the world around us. Hope, doubt, love, and anger are just a few examples of these themes, which I explore in ways you may never have considered and offer techniques to help you internalize. At no point do I sugarcoat my advice, but once you hit the pit of depression, you really don't need someone to tiptoe around the big issues. You want it laid out in front of you, for better or worse, so that you can manage your life and find happiness.

I wrote this book for anyone who has ever felt depressed, lost, and unable to just be happy. But I did not only write this book out of a desire to help others. As you can see in the book's dedication, I also wrote this for me. In my own recovery from depression, I knew that writing this book was necessary to avoid falling back into depression again. My many relapses with depression were due to ignoring the lessons I had learned whenever I got a little ahead in life. In Chapter 4, I will discuss your need to keep a journal. This book is my journal.

This book is the chronicling of the lessons I have learned through my own experiences, research, and discussions with others. It is my understanding of the world you and I were born into. It is the path that I took from those helpless days of sorrow, angst, anger, and doubt to moments of joy, appreciation, acceptance, and pride dispersed within a background feeling of calmness. What makes me qualified to write this book is that, like you, I have experienced depression. And like me, you will overcome it. So I write and dedicate these words both to you and to me.

There is a great deal in this world that I do not understand, but what I do know is that the ability to enjoy life is based on how you interact with this world. As a metaphor, consider the ability to drive a car. I do not personally understand the mechanics of how an automobile works, but I know that when I put the car in "drive," I move forward; when I put the car in "reverse," I move backward. My ability to operate the car is dependent solely on how I interact with it. Similarly, you only need to change how you interact with this world to truly let go of depression and find happiness.

You won't always get everything you want, plan for, or expect out of life. But no matter what you encounter, your only sense of control is in how you handle it. When you change your actions, you change your interactions with this world and consequently the way you feel; and that's really what we are concerned with: how you feel.

We all want to change the world,
but too often we allow the world to change us.

Chapter 2

Physically Induced Motivation

You can tell a lot about people by their appearance. You may have heard someone tell you that you look tired when you feel exhausted or been asked if anything was wrong simply based on your posture. The body is often a reflection of how you feel and, therefore, my question to you is: "When was the last time you smiled?"

I'm willing to bet that it's been a while. You may not even remember the last time you smiled as you might associate it with the last time you were truly happy and not know when that was. We are going to change all that together.

Just as your body reflects your emotional state, your body also affects your emotional state. In fact, one of the fastest and simplest ways of helping you feel better emotionally is changing the way you treat your body. Through certain daily actions, you can quickly give yourself the one thing you need most to both feel better and gain the ability to apply the concepts throughout this book into your life. That one thing you need right now is energy.

Energy is essential to life. It is the power needed to do anything and is commonly associated with feeling upbeat. Without energy, people hover on thoughts like suicide because death is purely an absence of energy. And when you have depression, you have a lack of energy; that is why it feels like dying.

The harmful cycle of energy loss that those with depression fall into starts with not maintaining healthy energy levels. When you have depression, the exhaustion you feel does not give you much motivation to work toward increasing your energy levels. By not trying to increase your energy, you then begin losing the energy you presently have and, therefore, have less enthusiasm to work toward improving your life. Essentially, your behavior makes you more and more depressed while making it harder and harder to acquire the energy necessary to be happy.

There are two ways to gain energy: physically and mentally. Both, if utilized, will give you motivation to help change behavior that may be keeping you depressed. This chapter will focus on ways to physically increase your energy, and later on in Chapter 5, we will discuss ways you can increase your energy using your mind. Because you may not have much energy right now and consequently little motivation to improve your life, the following are simple and straightforward methods that will help you improve your mood and increase your energy enough to follow the techniques throughout this guide.

Water

One of the most important things you can do to maintain high energy levels and overall health is drink water. Your body is made up of approximately 60-70% water.[1] It is found in your blood, muscles, and skin. Research has shown that even a two percent drop in body water reduces the brain's ability to function properly, leading to depressed emotions.[2] That means depression can be caused by dehydration![3]

Because there are so many different ways the body loses water, it is important to regularly replenish your body's water supply. You probably realize that you lose water in your body when you go to the restroom or by sweating, but you also lose water just by breathing. Think about when you breathe on glass, be it a window or mirror; you create a layer of vapor. If you run a finger over that vapor and then rub your fingers together, you can actually feel the moisture you exhaled in your breath. That means every few seconds when you exhale, you are losing body water.

When you wake up, you have been exhaling for hours without a single sip of water, making that a crucial time to hydrate. So each morning, as soon as you wake up, drink a tall glass of water. Then continue drinking water throughout the rest of the day. The average person loses approximately 10 cups (80 ounces) of fluid per day, making it essential to drink at least that much water every day.[4] Keep a water bottle with you at all times. This will make it easier to remember to keep drinking.

You will unlikely feel thirsty as often as you need to drink water, but thirst is actually a symptom of dehydration.[5] Once you are thirsty, your body has already been craving water for some time. Interestingly, the body sometimes induces hunger pains when it only needs fluids. Since hunger and thirst signals use the same hormonal alert system, one can often be confused for the other. So in addition to drinking at random times throughout the day, an important time to drink water is when you feel hungry. You may find that you weren't actually hungry but just in need of fluids.[6]

Water alone will not give you energy, but it is what carries nutrients to your cells that give you energy. It is one of the most valuable substances you can put into your body. In fact, you can't even live without water for more than a few days. Drinking water can also improve the appearance of your skin, flush toxins out of your body, keep you regular, and reduce your risk of disease.[7] These additional physical benefits often help build confidence and self-esteem because you can be proud of your body. So fill up your water bottle and drink from it throughout the day. In fact, right now is a great time to drink some water. Your ability to function depends on it.

<u>Dopamine</u>

In order to understand how to properly increase energy levels and feel good, it's essential to get a bit more scientific. There are several chemicals in your brain that physiologically affect your mood and motivation. Extensive research has focused on dopamine, serotonin, and melatonin. While serotonin and melatonin will be briefly discussed later in this chapter, I have found credible evidence to support dopamine as the chemical with the most significant link to combating depression and will, therefore, primarily focus on that.

Dopamine is associated with feelings of pleasure, love, concern for others, and reward sensations as well as attention and learning. A lack of this chemical in the brain, however, can reduce the ability to feel any pleasure or remorse in life. Sound familiar? Dopamine imbalances can lead to schizophrenia, Parkinson's disease, and yes, mood disorders like depression.[8] Using techniques to increase dopamine levels, physicians at Harvard Medical School have actually found good results reducing symptoms in medication-resistant depression.[9]

So the reasonable question is: "How can you increase your dopamine levels?" Positive social interactions, humor, massage therapy, and a number of different foods activate dopamine neurons.[8] The following sections are some of the easiest and most effective ways I have found to increase dopamine levels and overall energy when you are depressed.

Vitamins

Considerable evidence has shown that the addition of vitamins into the average diet can significantly improve one's health. While some studies may question the effectiveness and safety of certain vitamins, most experts agree that supplementing your diet with vitamins can be extraordinarily effective in providing you with physical and mental boosts of energy. Of course, when introducing any supplement into your diet, you should consult your doctor's advice if you are pregnant, lactating, or on prescribed medicine.

While eating your first meal of the day, you should take two specific supplements. One is a multi-vitamin; the other is 100mg of vitamin B complex. The multi-vitamin will help contribute to your overall health while the B complex will work directly toward turning food into mental and physical energy.[10] Vitamin B is associated with controlling stress levels, increasing energy, and stimulating the production of dopamine.[8, 11] I strongly believe that a great deal of depression is related to vitamin B deficiencies. In fact, medical research has shown some 70% of people to be vitamin B deficient, which could explain the abundance of people suffering from depression.[12]

It is true that the dosage of vitamin B that I am recommending is much higher than its daily value referenced on food labeling, but the daily values on food labels are not actually recommended intakes. They are "reference points" to help consumers get some perspective on their dietary needs.[13] When it comes to maintaining optimal health, including the energy needed to avoid depression, taking 100mg of vitamin B complex each morning along with a multi-vitamin can give you the boost you need to start feeling better.[14] Trust me, you will feel the difference.

When you buy your vitamins, I recommend buying timed release tablets. "Timed release" means that the vitamins will be absorbed into your body slowly. This will avoid a temporary quick burst of energy, and you will instead feel a constant stream of energy throughout the day. If you can't find vitamin B complex in 100mg dosages, you can purchase it in smaller dosages and load up to 100mg daily.

Be aware that taking these vitamins will cause your urine to turn a neon yellow color. Some people may claim that this means you are not absorbing the vitamins, but that is not entirely true. Your body is absorbing what it needs and you are peeing out the rest. So you are getting exactly the amount you need, no more, no less.[15] If, however, your urine is yellow but you forgot to take your vitamins, it means you're not drinking enough water.

B vitamins are water soluble, which means you can take your vitamins when you drink your water each morning. However, I have recommended taking them with your first meal to help ease absorption. Some people complain of upset stomachs when consuming vitamins with just water. Depending on how these vitamins react with your own body, you can choose to take them when you have your glass of water first thing in the morning or with food to reduce any queasiness.

In addition to taking a multi-vitamin and 100mg of vitamin B complex daily, there are several other supplements you can add into your diet to aid in motivation and reduce depression. Omega-3 fatty acids, bee pollen, rhodiola, SAMe, 5-HTP and St. John's Wart have been shown to have the beneficial effects required to raise your energy levels and brighten your mood.[16; 17] The last three, however, should be avoided if you currently are taking prescribed SSRI antidepressants, and bee pollen should be avoided if you have an allergy to bees.[18] While there are many different supplements that offer motivational boosts, the ones I encourage you to consume daily are 100mg of vitamin B complex and a multi-vitamin. This is a simple activity that can substantially help improve your health, reduce stress, stimulate dopamine production, and provide you the energy needed to put forth effort toward bettering your life.

Food

One of the primary ways you ingest vitamins and minerals is through the food you consume. What you eat and how much of it has a direct effect on your mental state. When depressed, people tend to handle food in two distinct manners. They either overeat or undereat. Both are harmful, and the way to determine if you fit into one of these categories is to consider how tired you get throughout the day. If you eat too much, your body diverts a lot of energy to breaking down the food. If you don't eat enough, you do not have enough fuel to provide adequate energy for the day.[19]

Many people with depression do not get hungry. If you fall into this category, remember to drink water. This should stimulate your body to crave food when it is needed. On the other hand, if you compensate for your depressed feelings by eating continually, drinking water will also reduce the need for food when you have eaten too much. Water is so fundamental to your well-being that drinking a glass of it can immediately tell you whether you need to eat or need to stop eating.

When you do start eating regularly, it is best to eat until you are approximately 80% full and then stop eating. This essentially means to stop eating when you feel the first signs of being full.[20] Eating slowly can significantly help you notice your body's signals of being full. In general, dietary guides, including the U.S. Department of Agriculture and the U.S. Food and Drug Administration, recommend the average person maintain a 2,000 calorie diet, consuming less than 65 grams of fat and 300 mg of cholesterol per day.[21]

There are several methods to avoid overeating when you feel the first signs of being full. Consider pouring water on the rest of your meal or giving the remainder of your meal to someone else, be it a friend or someone who is homeless. But the longer you sit with food close to you, the more likely you are to continue eating despite being full. When you sense that you are filling up, immediately move any food away from you; and drink water if you continue to feel hungry. You can function well on much less food than what many people consume as long as the food you are eating is healthy.

Food is the fuel for the mind and body. *What* you put into your body is just as important as *how much* food you put into your body. There are a number of foods that lead to reductions in energy and there are several foods that increase energy. The goal of eating is to get as much nutrition as you can from the food you consume. If your body is not getting the nutrients it needs, your brain will not function properly, which can translate into the psychological feelings associated with depression.

Good food choices that have energy-creating nutrients like vitamin B include the following:
Apples
Avocados
Bananas
Blue Berries
Citrus Fruits
Lentils
Oatmeal
Peanut Butter
Sardines
Spinach
Sweet Potatoes
Watermelon
Yogurt[22]

In general, foods high in protein (including protein shakes) will produce substantial energy that lasts throughout the day.

Foods high in protein include the following:
Beans
Cheese
Eggs
Fish
Meat
Milk
Nuts
Seeds
Soy
Yogurt[23]

Phenylalanine is an essential amino acid that is converted into the amino acid tyrosine in the body, which is what synthesizes dopamine. What this means is that increasing your phenylalanine levels can effectively treat depression. Phenylalanine can be found in foods such as meat, cottage cheese, and wheat germ. It is even in breast milk because of its importance in growth and energy. However, those who suffer from the rare genetic disorder phenylketonuria (PKU) should limit or, in some cases, avoid phenylalanine.[9]

Foods that lead to the production of dopamine include the following:
Apples
Beets
Blue-Green Algae
Celery
Cheese
Chicken
Cucumber
Duck
Eggs
Fish
Green Leafy Vegetables
Honey

Lean Beef
Pork Tenderloin
Sardines
Shellfish
Sweet Peppers
Tofu
Turkey
Watermelon
Wheat Germ[9; 24]

These are some good lists of foods that are healthy and will increase your energy; however, it's also important to be knowledgeable about foods that will reduce your energy levels. An ingredient to be aware of in food is salt (also known as sodium). Processed or pre-packaged foods, snacks, fast foods, and frozen dishes tend to be particularly high in salt content. Salt is vital to healthy living, but too much of it can dehydrate you. Since hydration is key in maintaining quality health and energy levels, try to avoid meals high in sodium or you may become tired shortly after eating. Your sodium intake should be limited to 2,400mg per day. Keep that in mind or you may become tired shortly after eating a high-salt meal or snack.[21]

One of the leading culprits of energy loss, however, is refined sugar. Unlike sugar found in fruits and vegetables, refined sugar can lead to reductions in energy and the deterioration of your body and mind. Refined sugar that is often found in candy, cookies, soft drinks, and many types of noodles undergoes a process that depletes it of nearly everything but the pure sugar before it is used to make these foods. The body, however, cannot digest and metabolize sugar properly unless proteins, vitamins, and minerals are present.[25] Since the refining process depletes the sugar of these resources, your body compensates for their absence by removing vital nutrients it has stored inside you (including vitamin B).[26]

One common misconception about refined sugar in regards to energy levels is the "sugar high." Refined sugar is a type of simple sugar, which doesn't require much breakdown by the body. It, therefore, reaches the bloodstream faster than many other foods, giving you an instant rush of energy. Too much of this sugar, however, causes the body to produce insulin to counteract its effects, which leads to a rapid drop in blood sugar. Low blood sugar means low energy. And this is the "crash" you may have heard about that can follow bursts of energy caused by eating refined sugar.[27]

As you limit your intake of foods made with refined sugar, you may experience withdrawal symptoms, including cravings, headaches, chills, and body aches. Refined sugar has addictive traits, and many dieticians actually consider it to be a drug because it acts more like a drug than food.[28] During this withdrawal period, consume more fruits and vegetables. The natural sugars in these whole foods can help to ease any withdrawal symptoms.[29]

Choosing what to eat is not always easy, but general guidelines will help you maintain a healthy eating lifestyle. Avoid foods that are fried, processed, made with refined sugar, and high in sodium content. Choose foods that are raw, steamed, stir fried, grilled, or baked. Eat lots of fruits and vegetables as well as whole grains and high-protein foods. The desire to eat junk food may overwhelm you at times, particularly when you are looking for any reason to be happy or just don't care about your well-being; but this is your chance to start feeling better. The healthier you eat, the more energy you will have; and in time, the better you will feel.

It's time to gain control over food rather than letting food control your happiness. Take the time to write down the food recommendations listed in this section and read the labels on the back of products you buy at the grocery store to learn what's in the food you plan to eat. Pay special attention to serving sizes, which may be smaller than the amount you intend to eat. Then take notice of how you feel in the hours after you eat different meals. Write down those patterns and consider them when debating what to eat the next time you are hungry. Make your own list of recipes and foods that give you energy. As you change your diet, you will notice the effects in your mood and energy levels; and you will realize that you truly are what you eat.

Drugs

I will not tell you not to do drugs. I am not going to point a finger at you and say what you should or shouldn't do based on societal standards. I don't believe that all prescription drugs should be praised, and I don't believe that all illegal drugs are bad. Everything in life can have a purpose, but if you are using drugs, it's essential that you ask yourself why you are making that choice.

If you are using drugs, examine the feelings that you get by your drug use both during and after you use them. Are you learning about yourself or just avoiding examining yourself? Are you helping your desire to improve your life in the long run or are you hindering it? Typically when people have depression and are regularly using drugs, they aren't helping themselves and would be better off by discontinuing their use. So take some time and consider the role that drugs play in your own life.

The reality is that most people who use drugs don't use them because drugs feel bad; they use drugs because they feel good. Sometimes when people feel numb, they use them just to feel something. Other times, when people hurt, they use them to dull their pain. Drugs can induce the feeling of a change in environment, but when it comes to depression, it is up to you to overcome it, not mask it.

For many people on the path to improve their lives, they see drugs as tools that allow them to think differently and, therefore, have important realizations about themselves and the world. While many drugs can offer the opportunity for realization, it's equally important to recognize that the point of a realization is to apply it to your life. Ask yourself how many times you would need to burn yourself on a hot stove before you realized that a red burner should not be touched. Similarly, consider how often taking drugs is necessary before the lessons learned while on them sink in. You shouldn't have to keep doing drugs indefinitely to regain any knowledge they have provided you. Take the lessons from your experiences with you into sobriety. Otherwise, a drug may have stopped being a tool and started becoming an escape.

One of the biggest problems for those who use drugs habitually is that drug addicts have malfunctions in their dopamine systems. Certain drugs like cocaine, heroin, opiates, alcohol, amphetamines, nicotine, and even caffeine briefly increase dopamine levels that lead to a temporary "high" but simultaneously damage the brain. The irony is that dopamine-stimulating drugs increase dopamine so intensely when you get high (making you feel good) that during sobriety there is not enough dopamine to disperse into the body consistently throughout the day (making you feel bad). This means that the more of these types of drugs a person uses to feel happy, the more difficult it becomes to be happy when not on those drugs.[9]

What's worse is that too much dopamine has been associated with addictive behaviors, increasing the physiological desire to use drugs frequently.[8] Furthermore, since dopamine leads to a feeling of pleasure, there is also the psychological desire to continue using drugs that spike your dopamine levels. Examples include when you hear about people "needing" their daily coffee, chasing a high, or craving a cigarette to calm themselves in stressful situations. Whatever the drug, these bursts of dopamine both risk your chances of addiction while causing you substantial sadness when the drug wears off.

It's my belief that one of the reasons withdrawal symptoms from drugs can be so intense is because of the mental attachment a person creates to the way the world appeared when high to the overwhelming difference of how it appears when sober. And that dramatic shift causes a deepening into sadness. The delusional realities drugs provide may offer a break from the pain of depression, but the end of the high (which always comes) brings the reverting change that the person loathes.

One controversial drug that remains in question is marijuana. Some evidence has shown that this drug actually has antidepressant properties. However, marijuana has also been associated with "amotivational syndrome" in which chronic users become apathetic, socially withdrawn, and function below their capacity.[30] Keep in mind that what is important at this point in your journey is gaining the motivation to overcome your depression. Even if marijuana brings a sense of relief from depression, it still can inhibit you from acquiring the motivation needed to improve your lifestyle. Considering that the drug is illegal in much of the world and your anxiety level would be dependent on a drug, there are much more effective ways to find happiness.

If you currently have an addiction to drugs, which you are unable to overcome on your own, an important step is contacting others for help. Friends, therapists, clinics, and online resources can all help you to stop using drugs. Feel free to call the National Substance Abuse Helpline at 1-800-662-HELP (4357), available 24 hours a day, which can direct you to local treatment centers.[31] Asking for help shows a great deal of strength on your part, and when you do reach out to others, you will find that there are people who care about your well-being even when you're not sure that you do. This may not be easy, but the first steps are always the most valuable. You are the one who has to say "yes" or "no" and endure the consequences.

There is no drug that cures depression; only a lifestyle change will help you overcome it. Any drug, be it illicit or pharmaceutical medication can be beneficial or harmful in your journey. However, no drug will help you find happiness in the long run if you aren't spending your time trying to improve the way you live. The real journey is not in the use of a drug but in the effort to better your life so that you don't need it.

Morning Activities

Each morning after you wake up and drink a glass of water, there are a number of other activities you can perform to increase your energy for the day. The next steps in your morning routine should include showering, stretching, getting dressed, and going outside.

Showering not only coats your body with the much-needed water you lost during sleep, but the change in environment from dry to wet signifies the start of the day. Many people take scalding hot showers that relax them, and some of these people even fall asleep in the shower. This is not the point of showering in overcoming depression. Instead, take a lukewarm shower. By taking a shower that is only mildly warm, you will spend less time in the shower and feel more awake when you dry off. Think about anytime the hot water has run out while taking a shower. The cold water with which you finished your shower very likely gave you immediate energy.

After you dry off, it's time to stretch. Stretching helps to move the energy you just acquired in the shower throughout your body. When you take a cold/lukewarm shower, you gain energy quickly; but you sometimes tighten up. By stretching, you open up your joints, muscles, and organs so that the energy you have acquired can enter each part of your body. You need your entire body to make it through the day. So channel that energy into the different parts of your body as you stretch all your limbs.

One particularly good stretch begins by standing with your legs straight and your feet about a foot apart from each other. Now reach up as high as you can, stretching your torso and arms up. Then, keeping your back straight and bending at the waist, let your torso come down in front of you slowly with your arms outstretched until you are dangling from your waist. Keep your legs straight and let your torso and arms hang loose in front of you. Swing your torso from side to side as your fingertips slowly get closer to the ground. Then, with your arms outstretched, slowly bring your torso back up and reach toward the sky, repeating the movement. Each time your torso hangs down from your waist, your hands should get a little closer to the ground. Don't worry about whether your fingers graze the ground; if you stretch regularly, eventually they will.

Other stretches include lying down and twisting your body at the waist. You can even stretch your tongue by sticking it out as far as you can in all directions. There are many stretches you can find out about online, from other books, or through the help of anyone who is knowledgeable in fitness. Try a variety of different stretches, but remember that stretching should be a slow process that takes at least 15 minutes. By rushing through stretching, you could pull a muscle; and you don't want that. The goal is to heal your body, not injure it.

Once you are done stretching, get dressed. Getting dressed tells your mind that you have work to do today and that energy is needed. Putting clothes on may seem like a given, but many people walk around in a robe or towel for far too long into the day. When you get dressed, it is also important to put on clean clothes. Wearing clothes that you've slept in, are stretched out, or are dirty can allow you to fall into a routine of not caring about yourself. If you are attempting to start each day fresh and clean, put on clothes that are fresh and clean. Unclean clothing will only make you want to go right back to bed.

Finally, it's essential that you spend some time outside every day. Air inside a home gets stale, and like the importance of putting on clean clothes, it is important to breathe clean air. It doesn't matter if you live in a polluted city or have an air purifier in your home; there is no substitute for fresh outside air. If it is raining, bring an umbrella out with you or stand under an awning. A walk outside will almost always help alleviate exhaustion. Even during the writing of this book, it was important that I took regular breaks to go outside and take a few deep breaths to gain the energy I needed to continue writing. It is my belief that you should breathe outdoor air approximately every two hours.

While you are outside, you will see two important energy stimulants; the first is the sun. The sun makes life possible. It distributes the energy it creates into nearly everything in this world. Even the food you eat that gives you energy got its energy from the sun.[32]

Getting enough sunlight during the day is related to the efficiency of many bodily functions. These include the production and release of chemicals and hormones that can affect your mood such as serotonin and melatonin, which I mentioned earlier in this chapter. In fact, some researchers have determined that light therapy may help to alleviate the symptoms of depression faster than antidepressant drugs. This lends understanding to why so many people have elevated moods in the summer months while depression numbers rise during the winter months. This phenomenon is called Seasonal Affective Disorder. What new research is finding, however, is that high amounts of sunlight exposure in summer can actually elevate moods for the upcoming winter. That means going outside in summer helps alleviate depression months later.[33]

The second stimulant you will notice outside each morning is other people. In addition to looking inside yourself, part of overcoming depression is looking outside yourself at others and how you interact with them. On an average day, when you look at someone who then looks back at you, chances are you quickly look down or away to avoid making eye contact. If you are in an elevator, you might look up instead. In either case, avoiding eye contact avoids creating the social connections you desperately need. Do you even know why we often don't look at other people in the eyes? Is it so that other people won't get offended? What is really so wrong with looking at another person?

Socializing can be very helpful with overcoming depression, and eye contact is one of the best ways to initiate a connection. When you make and hold eye contact with other people for more than a second, you may be surprised at how many of them say "hello" to you. Human contact is fundamental to survival and we are in constant need of connections.[34]

You may not always feel like seeing others, but creating a connection with someone else causes another person to care about your well-being even if you don't care about it. For someone else to say "hello," ask how you're doing, or even nod his/her head shows recognition and an interest in your life. And you may even find that those people's consideration for you causes you to begin caring about yourself. Those people you need for these connections can be found outside.

Exercise
Dopamine is a key chemical in affecting personal happiness, but the release of dopamine is only as good as the amount of dopamine receptors present in you. In your body, you have both dopamine and dopamine receptors; and the number of receptors determines how much dopamine can be utilized. Let's assume that your brain releases one ounce of dopamine into your body, but you only have enough receptors for half of an ounce. The extra half-ounce will not be absorbed. Fortunately, exercise has been found to increase your quantity of dopamine receptors.[35] And understandably, aerobic exercise has been shown as an effective treatment for depression.[36]

Part of the process of increasing your energy and feeling good about life will be dependent on incorporating exercise into your life. I have helped so many people get through swings of depression simply by encouraging them to get dressed, go outside, and run for a few minutes. That is why it was one of the first steps I recommended. Whether it's dance, basketball, yoga, or any other physical activity, I truly believe exercise is one of the best and healthiest ways to give you a quick lift when you are feeling down or exhausted. Combine exercise with fresh air and water, and you're on your way.

If you are just beginning to include exercise in your life after a lull or have never worked out, I advise making exercise a daily routine for two reasons. First, the more you exercise, the easier it will be to keep exercising because you get used to it. Second, by exercising daily, you help stimulate the creation of new energy so that you can start feeling better quickly.

Let's be real though; with a lack of motivation, it may be a stretch to start working out every day. Therefore, one method of getting your daily exercise is to take a brisk walk for 20-30 minutes when you first go outside each morning. However, when you have depression and are first starting to exercise, even 20 minutes can seem like a lot. So when you go outside, walk to the end of the block (or for one minute). If you feel like you can keep going, walk for another minute. Try running for a minute. Just a few minutes of jogging can substantially change the way you feel. The first step, however, is just getting outside. When you do, make the most of your time. Too many people spend the majority of their days indoors.

Getting outside your home to exercise is essential for all the reasons explained in the previous section, but it also helps to distance you from the couch, bed, refrigerator, television, and many other distractions that can cause you to lose your focus. However, if exercising inside your home is your only option, it is better than not exercising at all.

If you are finding that you do not have enough motivation to regularly exercise, a good technique is to join an exercise group or a class to stimulate your commitment to working out. Exercise groups and classes require obligation rather than exercising on your own, which requires dedication. And since low self-esteem is central to feelings of depression, obligations are typically easier to attend to than personal dedication. The added factor of a set time or having prepaid for a class may also encourage you to go.

Another technique that helps increase your motivation to exercise is listening to energetic music. Before heading outside your home to exercise, grab your music player and ear phones. The rhythm of upbeat music frequently helps people get energized to work out and makes the time spent exercising feel like it is flying by.

In addition to the energy and mood elevation that exercise induces, yet another benefit is physical appearance. As you get more in shape, you tend to feel prouder about your body, raising your level of self-confidence. By looking and feeling healthier, you also tend to live healthier, making healthier decisions about what you put into your body and how you spend your time.

Sleep and Relaxation
Much of this chapter has addressed methods of creating energy, but maintaining that energy is dependent on a good

night's sleep. Sleep is a lot like food in how it affects your energy levels; too much, too little, or the wrong kind will leave you depleted of energy. The right amount of sleep varies among age groups, but most adults need approximately 6-8 hours of sleep per night.[37] Less than this can make you tired throughout the day, and more can also make you tired because your body creates an attachment to sleep. In fact, both insomnia and over-sleeping have been linked to increased feelings of depression.[38] The best way to ensure you get this amount of sleep is to schedule and stick to a set bed time that is 6-8 hours before you need to be awake, and then set an alarm to wake you up. No one likes getting up to an alarm, but it will help with getting the right amount of sleep.

Personally, I recommend using an alarm that eases you into waking up. The start of your day should be relaxing, not jarring. Getting up can be difficult enough. If you use an alarm that makes you want to put a pillow over your head, you are going to start your day on a frustrated note. Instead, consider setting a radio alarm to a soft music channel to soothe your journey into the waking world. Maybe you have a favorite song that you can program into your phone as an alarm. There are even fancy alarms that wake you up with a slow ringing of soft bells or slowly illuminating lights. How you get up in the morning can have a significant effect on your energy levels for the rest of the day. So it's best that you find an enjoyable means of waking up rather than fighting your way into the day.

Even with an alarm, getting out of bed can sometimes be a difficult process. There are, however, several things you can do to make waking up easier. Sleep with a window open, avoid eating within two hours of going to bed, drink a glass of water before you go to sleep, turn up the heat in your room, and don't watch television or use the computer right before bed. It may also help to place a glass of water next to your bed so that as soon as you begin to wake up, you can take your first sip of water, enabling you to fully wake up before you even get out of bed. When you make these changes to your approach to sleep, the difference in waking up is literally like night and day.

In addition to the importance of how much sleep you get and how you wake up, you need to also get the right type of sleep: deep sleep. The athletic exercise you perform during the day will help you to sleep harder. Stress, on the other hand, will cause you to sleep lighter.[39] For many, meditation helps calm the mind. So if you are unable to fall asleep at night, try the following technique of meditating.

Technique: Meditation

Sit up with your back straight, your legs crossed, and your eyes closed. Place one hand on your belly and take a slow, deep breath, inhaling for four seconds through your nose. Make sure that as you breathe in, you feel your belly expanding. Hold this breath in your lungs for two seconds and then exhale your breath for six seconds through your mouth. After you do this, count the breath to yourself as *one*. Inhale again for four seconds, holding for two, and exhaling for six. Count this breath as *two*. Try following this breathing method until you get to ten breaths. If your mind wonders and you lose count, start again by counting your next breath as *one*. Don't get frustrated if this proves to be difficult as people who practice this meditation for years regularly lose count. When your mind wonders, don't judge yourself for wherever your thoughts take you. Instead, be mindful of the thoughts that come into your head and just breathe them out as you exhale, counting your next or first breath. Continue this until you realize that you are relaxed. Then lie down and go to sleep.

———

There are several different ways to meditate, but the most important part of this technique is that you focus on your breathing. By focusing on the inhalation and exhalation of your breath, you quiet the chatter inside your head. You concentrate on the flow of your breath and let go of the many negative thoughts that accompany depression.

For so many of us, we don't take quiet time for ourselves because it feels uncomfortable. We're so used to hearing the voice in our heads shouting about what we should and shouldn't do that sitting in silence both amplifies the volume in our own heads and makes us feel as though we should be focusing on improvement rather than just relaxing. While there are certainly times when we need to explore our lives through thought, the effort and ability to be calm in silence eases your worries; and that *is* improvement.

Meditation can offer many benefits to those who use it. In fact, meditation is often recommended to help people overcome panic attacks commonly associated with depression. When you experience a panic attack, you take rapid, shallow breaths that can cause hyperventilation. By practicing controlled, deep breathing through meditation, however, you can correct your breathing and help prevent panic attacks from occurring in the future.[40]

Review

These methods of choosing wisely what you put into your body and what you do with it physically throughout each day do not take much time but can significantly help increase the amount of energy you have. They may even provide you with more time during your day by allowing you to get things done quicker with your newfound energy.

All this is a lot to remember. So make a list and post it where you will see it every morning. Maybe it is best in your bedroom, next to your alarm clock, or in your bathroom. You decide.

Each Day:
Wake Up with an Alarm
Drink Water (including first thing in the morning)
Take Vitamins
Shower
Stretch
Get Dressed
Go Outside
Exercise
Eat Right
...and Sleep

These are the primary physical activities that will help you create and maintain high energy levels necessary to make changes to your life. They do not necessarily need to occur in the listed order, but each step can help heighten the amount of energy you have and consequently improve the way you feel. Other energy raising ideas that you may want to incorporate into your life may include putting new insoles in your shoes, using a juicer to make fresh juice, opening up your windows during the day to let fresh air into your home, getting a massage, performing nasal irrigation, playing with puppies at the pound, going to a park, doing hand stands, and putting on happy music. Monitor which behaviors provide or reduce energy for you personally, and use that information in your daily life.

The hardest part of these physical activities will be initiating them. Force yourself to make the effort. They will become easier for you over time and prove worthwhile as you gain the energy needed to pull you out of your funk and into the life you want to live.

The journey out of depression is uphill,
but it's a hell of a view when you reach the top.

Chapter 3

The Value of Results

Now that you are taking the time to treat your body better, you may be starting to feel some improvement in your overall well-being. Therefore, it's time to introduce some important concepts that often plague those regularly disappointed with life.

We are frequently led to believe that there is something more we must achieve in this life to be happy, and once we do that, things will be alright. But while many people may believe that they will be identified by what they have gained or lost, rarely do those past experiences make those people happy now. This is because when it comes to your personal feelings of joy, you identify yourself less with what you have done or not done with your life and more with what you are currently doing with your life.

People, however, still strive for results that they believe will make them complete, whether it is marriage, children, an educational degree, or a particular job. People seek results as a determination of who they are because they believe certain results represent success and suggest something definitive about their lives to themselves and to others. They believe that once they reach their goals, they will no longer have to work as hard for happiness because they will have achieved what they desire.

What these people are forgetting is that once their aspirations have been met, they then still have to live with them. For example, some might believe that once they get married, their relationship will have reached its fullest expression of love. Once married though, they discover that the relationship takes constant work to keep it going strong. It takes just as much effort to maintain the existence of results as it does to achieve the results in the first place. Sometimes it takes more effort to maintain them. Suddenly, an accomplishment can feel like an obligatory burden and a reason to be depressed.

The truth is results alone will not bring you happiness; only a continuous effort to do what makes you proud of yourself every day will do that. I am by no means implying that results are not important. If you never achieved results, you would eventually stop making an effort. But while the feeling of accomplishment is very rewarding, results are never the end of a journey. They are the midway point between everything you do to achieve the results and everything you do with them.

It takes effort to get a result, but if you don't follow it up with more effort, the result is nothing more than a title. And how valuable are titles? People think they hold importance, but they aren't nearly as important as what it takes to maintain those titles. People long for titles, such as boyfriend, girlfriend, president, doctor, etc. However, it is the action that makes you who you are, not the title. Titles typically only serve the ego, and without consistent effort to maintain them, titles eventually lose all clout.

For many, the thought of not achieving the title they desire is actually what stops them from doing what they would do *if* they had that title. For example, you might want to be a great basketball player. Great basketball players practice daily. You might think that you would practice daily if you were a great basketball player, but you don't regularly practice because you don't hold that title. However, the way you become a great basketball player is by practicing daily. The title doesn't dictate the behavior. The behavior dictates who you are, title or not. Whether or not you play for an NBA team is beside the point. If your goal is to be a great basketball player, by doing what one does, you become that.

This is true for everything in your life. You become respectful by giving respect rather than making it a conditional act. You become happy by doing what makes you feel good rather than finding something that makes you happy. You become identified by any action you choose to pursue in life, but the results you do or do not achieve don't represent you; you represent yourself by what you do with those results or without them.

The delusion that happiness is based on results incorrectly convinces so many people that they will never be happy. They become disappointed when the results they seek don't materialize and frustrated when the results they get don't quell their depression. The problem, however, resides not in their ability to be happy but in their belief of what will make them happy.

Results are not only a problem when sought as a means to an end but also when used as an excuse. Many people who are depressed label themselves with psychological disorders or permanent characteristics to avoid taking responsibility for why they feel the way they do. They see their inadequacies as simply the results of who they are. But let's be honest; holding a label over oneself may excuse negative feelings or behavior, but it doesn't make you feel any better. You still encounter the same problems. The only difference is that you have convinced yourself that you can't do anything about your life. When you place a label on yourself, you believe you are the way you are and little can be done to change that.

Do not mistake my implication. You may actually have a mental or physical condition that requires therapy, but it's essential that your diagnosis not be used as a reason for your depression. Rather, your depression should be used as a reason to do something about your condition.

The effort you make in life toward doing anything always indicates the direction in which you are moving. When you focus on your depression, you're looking right at it. It can be overwhelming and naturally depressing. But when you focus on the effort you make toward bettering your life, you're no longer facing your depression; you're seeing your energy. And that's how you move forward, making your depression, which is the result of your past, simply a step in the journey of your life.

The Value of Effort

Everything you do involves effort and it is that effort that makes you proud or disappointed with the life you are living. There may or may not be a point when your life ends that you get to look back on it all and say, "I achieved what I wanted" or "I didn't." However, you look at your life all the time, and that is when you get to ask yourself the question: "Am I doing what's important to me?" Your answer to that question is linked to whether you are happy or depressed.

Your feelings are most affected by what you are doing with your life because both your feelings and your effort always exist in the present. Results, on the other hand, only show up briefly in the present but spend most of their time as goals or memories. It is merely the way you interpret and react to past results or future ambitions that affect you today.

Your effort, however, is also subject to your interpretation. You may look down at your effort, critiquing yourself for not doing enough, not doing a better job, or not having started your effort earlier; but every moment is a new chance to start over. In this moment, if you feel as though your effort isn't enough, put forth more. It's as simple as that. But you have to consider whether your view of your effort is actually a view of your results. Are you looking at what you are doing and critiquing your actions or are you looking at what you haven't accomplished and judging your effort based on that? Rather than trying to make things perfect, do your best and don't worry about the results. If you can't find value in the journey of what you're doing, do something else because you'll spend most of your time unhappy otherwise.

Whether or not you look back at what you have and haven't done, the past is never definitive. Your behavior right now is what defines you. Think about it; you are reading a book about bettering your life, and in some small way, can't you feel that you are learning? Your actions right now are identifying the type of person you are. You are someone in pursuit of a better life. Regardless of how much you have accomplished yet or what challenges you may face, you are what you do in life; and how well you succeed at what you do is less important than the effort you put forth. This is because in life, you cannot often see the end result of your actions; but you always know your intentions. And your effort to live a specific way is evidence to yourself of your commitment to who you are choosing to be.

You need to commit more of the type of behavior that represents the type of person you want to be. When you don't, you experience feelings like guilt and depression. In fact, anytime you feel bad, you can ask yourself what you were just doing or thinking about and you will immediately know areas of your life you need to change. When you understand that the way you live your life identifies you, you gain the freedom to make that change on a whim. You can pursue a new direction in life without the effects of the past holding you back. While some people may continue to judge you based on past experiences if that is all they know of you, you will notice changes in yourself right away.

Most people, however, do not view those they know strictly based on their pasts. Rather, statements about someone's past are typically followed up with what that person is doing now. For example, instead of saying that a person had a hard life, people will often explain that the person had a hard life and how he/she has handled it. Results rarely define you as much as you might think they do. You write your own life in the present.

True happiness only comes from the way you live. Not talent, intellect, nor status has as great of an impact on your life as effort. But it is not just your effort that gives your life value; it is your appreciation of your effort.

Altering Your Past
When you make a mistake, you lose something. It may feel like a loss of freedom, a loss of a relationship, or possibly a loss of self-pride; but what you truly lose is the way of life you envisioned yourself having. It is changed in some way, and it

is that feeling of change from what you foresaw to something different that causes you to view past actions as mistakes.

Many people who are depressed often look back at the past as a better way of life. They remember how their lives used to be and how they subsequently wish their lives were now. And in making the comparison between a better-former life and a worse-present one, they often see their past actions and experiences as having caused problems for them now. They look back for reasons when they should be looking at how to improve their current circumstances. They see the results of the past instead of the effort they could make in the present. They think thoughts like, "If I could only go back and change what happened, everything would be better now." The inability to correct the mistakes of the past makes many people see their resulting present circumstances as equally unchangeable, which makes them feel as though they are doomed to a life of consequential depression.

But what if there was a way to change your past? If you could change the past, you could consequently improve the way you feel now. Well, changing the past may not be as impossible as you think.

Take a moment and consider any one of your memories. There are certainly details about that memory that are fuzzy. You experienced the memory from a particular perspective, and over time, bits and pieces have become less important than the overall theme of what took place. Now consider that each day thousands of people argue in courtrooms about the accuracy of memories just like yours. Attorneys question what took place in the past, and witnesses argue and believe that events occurred in a variety of different ways.

These situations suggest that the past is not as concrete as people often perceive it to be. Rather, the past is a perception. It is only as definitive as people experience it in the present. What you remember and how a past experience affects you today define what happened in your life. The past is only a story of why the present is the way it is.

So if the past is not as specific as we perceive it to be but is a personal experience that must be recalled, changing the past is as simple as changing how the past affects you. By altering the impact of the past on your present circumstances, you effectively change the past.

Say, for example, you had a fight with someone in the past that left you both not speaking to each other. The event might stand out as an important moment in your past. If you then reached out to that person and mended the breach in your relationship, the effects of that fight would not be as significant. You might even forget about the fight over time as your past is only what you remember and its present effect on you. As your perspective changes, so does your view of history.

Of course, you cannot literally change the past. What has transpired is over and you cannot go back and change it, but you can change how the past affects you, which is what really matters. You can act now to make amends for mistakes. How the past affects the present and subsequently the future is not set. The past is constantly changing by how you experience it in the present.

You might believe that this view of the past is pointless because you aren't literally changing the past; you are only changing the way the past affects you. But you have just as much control over the past as you do over the future. When you act now to affect the future, you are putting forth effort to get you to a point that you believe will make you happy. There is no certainty you will reach your goal, but your effort increases the probability that you will achieve the feeling you seek. Similarly, when you act now to change the impact of the past, you are working toward creating a life that makes you feel good. Your effort does not guarantee any physical change to the past, but it likewise increases the probability that you will feel happy based on your action. In this sense, the past and the future are nearly identical. We just tend to approach them differently.

What matters is not what has happened, but how you act now in relation to what has happened. Therefore, you are not bound to your past. Rather, your past is bound to your perspectives on your life in the present. The standard belief in this world is that by acting now, you cannot alter your past;

but it is your actions now that affect your past very significantly.

This is an important concept because the way you view your past's impact on your life is central to your ability to move forward. Your memories affect how you think, feel, and act. And your connection to the past may be inhibiting you from appreciating what you have in the present or going after what you want in the future. By accepting that your past is not an unchangeable experience that defines your present circumstances, you gain the ability to confront your past and eliminate its control over your life.

You have made mistakes in life. We all have. The truth is you will make mistakes in the future as well, but mistakes do not define you; how you work to correct them determines who you are. On the flipside, you may have been honored for past achievements; but whether you put the talent you used to accomplish those achievements into action now is what makes you a success or a has-been.

You may feel as though your life is a mess and yearn for better days from the past, but I assure you that your life is not worse off than it used to be. You just lost your way. You forgot how to appreciate. Nothing is perfect, but that doesn't change the fact that there are some wonderful things in this world; and you're one of them. You realize your own value when you are proud of yourself, and the way to take pride in yourself is by pursuing what is important to you and leaving behind what doesn't matter.

Doing what is important does not necessarily mean doing something extravagant. It doesn't mean changing the world. Doing what is important *to you* merely means doing what you value. This could be as simple as helping a friend, learning a new hobby, or working for a degree. The importance of anything you have or do in your life is determined by you.

Finding your way is more important
than reaching your destination.

Chapter 4

Predicting the Future

Examining and changing the effects of the past on your life is important in overcoming depression. It allows you to let go of what is gone, making the most of what is here. However, many of us make bad decisions because we don't know what our decisions will lead to in the future. Obviously, having insight into the future would provide anyone a great advantage, particularly those who feel their lives are destined for hardship. Well, through careful examination of your life, the apparent impossibility of looking into the future becomes somewhat possible.

Just as the past is not as definitive as most of us perceive it to be, the future is not as random as it might seem. A quote that is the basis for predicting the future came from George Santayana who said, "Those who cannot remember the past are condemned to repeat it."[1] I mentioned early on that people often encounter the same type of experiences repeatedly, only with different circumstances. The reasoning for this is because people's approaches to life typically don't change over time. Their approaches don't change because they don't recognize their past as an indication of the future. They see every situation as independent from every other. But while you are not bound to your past, your ability to bring about or avoid the reoccurrence of experiences is dependent on your ability to remember the big picture of what has happened in the past. This is because humans follow patterns.

A pattern is simply the repetition of a cause and its effect; certain approaches lend themselves to specific consequences.

People often put themselves in similar situations repeatedly with the same end result, failing to learn lessons from their experiences, both good and bad. They become attached to certain thoughts, behaviors, and feelings even if they are uncomfortable.

While it may seem undesirable to make the same mistakes repeatedly, patterns are not always bad. They are the reason psychology works and are essential to survival. For example, you have learned from your experiences with fire that if you get too close to it for too long, you will get burned. If it weren't for patterns, everything you do would require conscious thought and consideration. By and large, patterns keep you safe and enable you to do everything from tying your shoes to holding a conversation. They exist to help you integrate with this world, understanding on a subconscious level how your actions affect your experiences. You will now just need to use your patterns more effectively by being aware that they exist.

The future is about possibility, which means anything can happen; but it is also about probability, which is based on your past experiences. If the same type of behavior has led to the same results several times, it's likely that repeating the behavior again will generate the same outcome as it has on previous occasions. For example, if every time you had an alcoholic drink, you reacted by drinking several drinks, it's likely that having a drink in the future will result in you getting drunk.

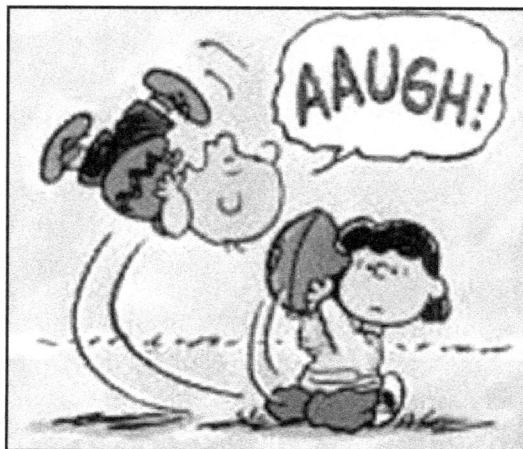

I recall Charles Schulz's "Peanuts" comic strip in which Charlie Brown would regularly attempt to kick a football that Lucy was holding for him. At the last minute, Lucy would swipe the ball away, causing Charlie Brown to fly through the air and come crashing down on his back.[2]

Charlie Brown's fall is both a result of Lucy's patterns and his own. Lucy's pattern is pulling the football away when Charlie runs to kick it, and Charlie's pattern is attempting to kick the ball when Lucy is holding it. Until one of them breaks character, Lucy will continue to deceive Charlie, and he will continue getting hurt. In your own life, you may play one of these characters. However, by recognizing both sets of patterns, you can make the choice to change your actions in relation to your surroundings to avoid impending hardships.

Assume that Charlie Brown's attempt to kick the football represents your attempt to tackle an issue in your own life, be it self-serving or just to be nice. Lucy pulling away the football will represent being taken advantage of, some sort of frustration, or failure. The natural question is how many times should you (or Charlie Brown) make an attempt to tackle the issue (or kick the football) before giving up. The answer to how many tries anyone should put forth in a repeatedly unsuccessful endeavor is:

> Once you notice the signs of a pattern, make one final attempt to confirm you have actually identified a pattern. If your final attempt results in the same general reaction, confirming a pattern exists, it is then up to you to consciously change your future behavior to effectively change future outcomes.

While you have a duty to treat people with respect (I will explain why later on), one of those people you need to give respect to is you. You don't need to sacrifice your self-respect at the expense of giving others respect. If patterns suggest that a situation is likely to end up causing you pain and hardship, you are better off focusing your energy on areas that patterns suggest will bring about joy and fulfillment.

At times in your life, you may just have to walk away from what you really want if patterns have shown that achieving your desire is nothing more than a fantasy. You may be used to aiming for the football and falling on the ground. And if so, you have to make the conscious decision not to go after the football when a Lucy in your life is holding it. There are better things in life to aim for.

Just as we do not always remember the past exactly as it happened, predicting the future is not a perfect science. Varying factors might cause someone's response to you to suddenly be different from pattern behavior of the past. This is what people often hope for when repeatedly pressing issues with others. But while anything is possible, recognizing patterns is generally reliable and can save you a lot of energy and hardship.

What you will often find when you change your patterns is that you have different experiences. You then must react to the new situations in the best way you can. You may find that when you change your pattern responses to others, their pattern responses toward you will change. However, these reactionary changes may only be temporary. They may be due to people not getting what they want from you rather than a genuine reconsideration of your feelings.

Consider these changed reactions to be one-time opportunities. For example, if Charlie Brown decided not to kick the football when Lucy held it for him, she might respond by promising that she would not pull the football away anymore. If she then broke her promise, committing to her original plan, Charlie Brown could dust himself off and walk away knowing he tried his best. The fact is that when you give your all, you no longer have any more energy to put forth on an endeavor.

In this example, not only were both characters' patterns identified; but Charlie Brown deciding to change his pattern was confirmed as a wise decision. Unfortunately, these confirmations typically take time to be seen. Throughout your life, it will be up to you to keep your eyes open for both beneficial and damaging patterns.

By recognizing patterns in your own life, you can clearly see how you are likely to react to future situations and what will likely result from your own actions. Many of us try to get others to change their behavior, but when it comes to your interactions, the most direct path to change is changing yourself. You play an important role in what happens in your life. People rarely realize that they are repeating ineffective habits, but a closer examination at one's life clearly displays that the responsibility for a person's position in life lies centrally with that individual. Even if you feel like the victim of unfair circumstances, repetitious experiences are rarely coincidental. They are almost always the result of your own patterns in relation to others' patterns.

Perhaps you feel like you have the worst luck in dating and that everyone you've ever dated has cheated on you. It's essential to consider that it may be the result of something you're doing, possibly even related to what you look for in a potential love interest. Until someone changes his/her behavior, situations are likely to repeat. However, because so many people and situations will come in and go out of your life, most of the time it will be on you to make change.

It is not so much the events in your life that have shaped you. Rather, it is the way you have experienced those events and how you reacted that made you who you *were*. It is your continuation to react the same way to similar events that makes you who you *are*. By looking at your past to determine your future, you can change your behavior in the present to create a whole new reality.

Why We Create Negative Patterns

If pattern behavior can lead to the repetition of negative experiences, why do we create negative patterns? There are three reasons. The first reason is the opposite of remembering the past; it is simply memory loss. People often say hindsight is 20/20, meaning you can clearly look back on a situation and see what you should have done rather than what you did. However, people only say this when the results of their decisions are contrary to their intentions. Hindsight is not 20/20; rather, it is blind. In any past experience, there were reasons you made the decisions you did. It is the failure to remember those reasons after an experience has occurred that makes memory loss a reason for the existence of negative patterns.

When you are upset and look back at circumstances that led to an undesired experience, you are unable to put yourself back in the mindset you were in at that time. Instead of connecting with your original thoughts and feelings that prompted your behavior, you instead connect with who you are now and wish you had acted differently.

Memory loss, however, works both ways. Those who forget their initial feelings that influenced their actions also forget their feelings that resulted from their actions. When a similar situation later arises, people tend to forget how they felt initially in the original situation as well as the pain they felt as a result of their actions. Thus, they consequently act similar to how they did originally and are consequently creating a reactionary pattern in response to the situational pattern being presented to them. Instead of looking at the past to predict the future, people focus so much on what they want (kicking the football) that they forget that every time they go after that desire, they fail (having the football swiped away from them).

The second reason we create negative patterns is due to something called inside perspective. This is the concept that when you are immersed within a situation, you fail to see the bigger picture.

It is usually not until someone is out of a situation or relationship that he/she can look back on it with a sense of clarity and reason. Just the same, many people may be in bad relationships, which everyone but them seems to realize. This often happens because those people focus their attention on the details of their experiences instead of considering third-party points of view.

Imagine you are standing in a square room facing one of the four walls. You could accurately describe the details of that one wall but would have little understanding of the other surrounding walls of the room. However, if you stepped out of the room and looked in from above, you would see the room as a whole and be better able to describe all the walls in the room. Similarly, when you are involved in any one of a variety of circumstances, you may tend to focus on minutia (one wall) rather than the bigger picture (the entire room).

People see what they want to see. They tend to focus on the details of situations, believing that the circumstances they are presented are different from past experiences. The truth is that every situation is different from every other situation when you consider locations, people's feelings, and various other contributing factors. The underlying issue, however, often is the same in many of these cases and, therefore, different situations end up the same way.

It is necessary for you to understand that patterns are not always dependent on the stimulus. What I mean by this is that circumstances do not typically influence one's behavior. Rather, it is often what someone wants to get out of a situation that causes the repetition of behavior and consequently the repetition of outcome. Charlie Brown wanting to kick the football may have little to do with actually kicking a football. It may come from the desire to be admired were he able to kick the ball well. The details of the situation are essentially irrelevant. Whether he was presented the opportunity to shoot a basketball or any other challenge, it is the interpretation of the event that holds significance for Charlie Brown.

The final and most common reason we create negative patterns is familiarity. Every living creature in this world seeks security, something that cannot exist in unfamiliar surroundings. The patterns people create may not be enjoyable, but often they are familiar. Even if something familiar is unpleasant, it feels more secure than the unknown. So if you repeat the same actions in your life and are frequently involved in the same type of situations, you eventually become familiar with those experiences, making you feel secure and giving you a (sometimes false) sense of comfort.

This is a major reason why many people remain in abusive relationships or with jobs they hate. Their repetitive engagement in a situation breeds an attachment of familiarity to it. They may consciously loathe their predicament, but the basic human need for security subconsciously draws these people to it again and again. And over time, their experiences begin to feel normal. They fail to see that they are actually reinforcing negative patterns in their lives. Instead, all they see is themselves putting forth effort and experiencing undeserved hardship.

Those with depression often feel like life regularly beats them down and that it is normal for them to suffer. This is also because of familiarity. Even the repetition of emotions creates a sense of familiarity. The regularity at which people place themselves in stressful situations leads to the regularity at which those people feel bad. On a conscious level, they want their circumstances and the way they feel to change; but subconsciously, they are seeking out experiences that make them feel bad because *that* is familiar. And in a way, that familiarity is comforting. That familiarity, however, is also inhibiting them from recognizing the urgency or even the possibility of changing their lives. They believe that their hardships are the result of coincidence rather than their own predictable behavior. Familiarity equals security, which equals comfort; but sometimes it's just a form of complacency.

Without the understanding that you have a distinct role in what you experience, you won't take the time to analyze that role. Whether it is your perspectives or actions, your part in your life is substantial. In fact, your role *is* the effort you will hear me discuss throughout this book.

People rarely take a step back and look at situations, both in how they are treated and how they are acting in accordance with that treatment. However, taking a step back is exactly what is needed to evaluate a situation and check for patterns in both yourself and in others.

Why We Maintain Negative Patterns

Now that you understand why we create negative patterns, the obvious subsequent question is why don't we break them. There are likewise three reasons for this. The first reason is purely that many of us do not recognize that patterns exist in our lives. We may feel the same bad feelings repeatedly, but we don't consider why we feel those ways. We do not see our own roles in causing ourselves to feel bad. Rather, we blame outside events for having caused negativity in our lives.

Typically people only notice the characteristics of a pattern when they repeatedly encounter the same negativity in "coincidentally" similar circumstances. But even when this cycle is recognized, the understanding that a *personal* pattern exists is rarely confessed. You might question, "Why does this always happen to me?" Or you might go further and think, "I attract negativity." But even then, there is no exploration done into how your actions bring about the circumstances you encounter. You merely blame others or coincidence, meanwhile believing that you can't do anything about your predicament. Without recognition and subsequent exploration, understanding, and modification of your patterns, you will encounter the same situations and experience the same emotions throughout the rest of your life.

The second reason we allow our negative patterns to continue is due to laziness. In fact, for many, laziness is a pattern. When a pattern of laziness exists in someone who has other negative patterns, that person has little energy to make the effort to overcome those negative patterns. Changing your life requires effort and commitment. If you don't consistently put forth the effort to improve your life, it won't improve. You will encounter the same experiences repeatedly and remain unhappy.

The last reason negative patterns are maintained is the same reason why human beings seek the security of familiarity: fear of the unknown. The possibility of something harmful happening stops people every day from pursuing what they desire. Even if leaving one situation for another could lead to positive experiences and a happier life, many people are unwilling to give up what they are used to for circumstances that will require adjustment. What is ironic about this perspective is that life is constantly changing anyway. While patterns suggest the likelihood of certain future events, anything can change in an instant.

Unless change is subtle or forced upon people, they are typically unwilling to shake their own trees. For many, the comfort in familiarity, which may even be an uncomfortable situation, often appears better than an uncertain future because of the fear that it could be worse than what they have now. They view any pain they are currently experiencing as manageable because they have learned to live with it. Even though a change in circumstances would probably be beneficial, the fear of not being able to manage something different creates an attachment to a currently harmful situation that one day may just become unmanageable.

When people have survived difficult times, they tend to think that they can deal with anything. Too often this is misinterpreted to mean that they can withstand suffering rather than using that strength to change their circumstances. The truth is what doesn't kill you only makes you stronger *if* you learn from the experience.

Whether it is not recognizing existing patterns, laziness, or fear that maintains one's negative patterns, the underlying theme of why people maintain those patterns is nearly always disguised with excuses. It is much easier to point a finger at why you don't have the life you want than to look within and put forth the effort to make a change. Sometimes the excuse is a lack of time to make change. Other times, people convince themselves that they don't really want change. Maybe they blame another person, the past, or their own characteristics. Whatever the excuse, dissatisfaction with your life is evidence that you're not dealing with your circumstances as well as you think. Life cannot simply be about surviving. It must be about living.

Keeping Your Journal

Before you can go about changing your behavior, you have to be able to identify existing patterns in your life. The best way to recognize patterns in your life is to get a journal and write in it every day. This can be a nice journal bought at a bookstore or simply a notebook. Do not hesitate to buy one though. If you don't have time to get a fancy journal soon, use a cheap notebook, which you can get at any drugstore. The book is not important, just the writing.

Throughout this guide, there will be several references to your journal and many techniques that involve writing in it. Therefore, it is very important that you get your journal immediately as it will play an important role in your recovery and sustaining happiness thereafter.

In addition to aiding in the techniques throughout this guide, your journal will serve three primary purposes. The first purpose is to identify patterns in your life. A journal will contradict memory loss because it is documentation of what has happened: your initial behavior, the situation, your reaction, and the outcome. By writing down and reading your actions and experiences, you will begin to see what you are doing that is causing yourself problems and what you are doing to solve your problems.

The second purpose of your journal will be to give you an outlet to write down what is going on in your life, including your actions, feelings, and thoughts. By writing your daily life down, you will be able to separate yourself from the intensity of life. You can release your feelings onto a page as opposed to just experiencing them in your head. You will then be able to later read over your experiences from different perspectives as your mood changes. This ability to shift your perspective of an experience will dramatically reduce the intensity of how past events make you feel because you end up looking at situations from all sides. This can help tackle some of the pitfalls of inside perspective.

The third purpose is actually a bonus for you. By writing in your journal now and into the future, it will become your personal story of how you overcame depression and found happiness. It will be a valuable resource later to avoid falling back into depression by reminding you of the tendencies that led you down that road and the tools you used to improve your life.

Keeping a journal makes you more consciously aware of how you are spending your days. Many people are passing through their lives without acknowledgement of the way they are feeling, what they are thinking, or what they are doing. A journal forces you to take time to review your life regularly by writing about it. Documenting your experiences, feelings, and realizations will give you the ability to recognize the impact of all these on your life so that you can keep it all in perspective.

Make sure you write in your journal consistently. No matter how tired you are or exhausted from a situation, writing in your journal will help you to compose your thoughts, seeing the big picture of your experiences, recognizing patterns, and understanding the decisions you make. When it comes to writing in your journal, what is most important is that you write in it after events, conversations, or thoughts that affect you deeply. Situations that you interpret as good or bad are the ones that personally impact you the most and will be valuable in recognizing your patterns of behavior and patterns of resulting circumstances.

Technique: Stimulating Your Writing

Writing in your journal will play a major role in getting to know yourself and the world around you. Occasionally though, you might feel too depressed or agitated to write in your journal; and at other times, you may feel as though you have nothing to say. If you're having trouble writing, the following methods may help get you going:

1.) Write whatever comes to mind whether it seems journal-worthy or not. Write about your day and what you wanted to accomplish. You can even literally write "I don't have anything to say" over and over until your mind wonders to other things for you to write about. By writing whatever pops into your head, it is likely that your writing will eventually direct itself to unresolved and important issues in your life.

2.) Select a random word to write about. The word can be any word at all. Open a dictionary if it helps or point to a random word in this book. Then write about what that word means to you or what experiences or thoughts it brings to mind. Again, your writing will likely begin addressing those issues that are engaging your focus.

3.) Read over some of your writing. When you review your own thoughts and experiences, you may uncover information about yourself. Write about whatever your past writing brings to mind. Write down questions you have about yourself or possible patterns you think may exist.

Whether you use one of these methods to begin writing, use your own method, or are able to pick up a pen/pencil and begin writing with ease, what matters is that you write. Writing will bring out information you might not have considered about your life. Most of us cannot write as fast as we think. Therefore, writing can force you to slow down your thoughts in order to keep up. When you slow your mind, you are able to really take notice of yourself rather than racing through your thoughts and consequently not addressing your concerns.

―――

While writing in your journal can bring out important information about your life, a journal is only as useful as your commitment to writing in it *and* reading it. Therefore, I recommend writing in your journal daily and reading it weekly. This way, you're not just writing about your life; you're learning about it. Pick a day that fits best into your schedule to read over your thoughts and experiences that you have documented. Then write the day you selected on the cover of your journal so you remember to read back over your writing on that day.

I have personally looked back on old journals in which I foretold the future with incredible accuracy because I identified patterns in my writing. However, it was my failure to read my journals and address the patterns I identified that allowed them to repeat in my life for far too long. Don't let this happen to you. You may be writing notes now that will help you determine the future and avoid unnecessary pain.

Your journal is a place for you to be honest with yourself and freely write exactly what you experience and feel. So keep your journal in a safe place. You may even want to keep it with you at all times, which can help you to quickly reference your past or describe a new experience.

Identifying Patterns in Your Life

Patterns become negative when they repeatedly lead to pain and suffering. These are the patterns that must be broken. You will need to reexamine how you are approaching and responding to the situations you encounter and take notice of what actions and reactions are leading to personal suffering. Your behavior may not seem like it should cause you to feel bad, but that may just be what is happening. Charlie Brown wanting to kick a football is not wrong. However, when you include the surroundings, which may be places, people, or emotional states, the activity leads to an undesired result that is deepening his depression.

Just as your behavior may not seem to be wrong, your circumstances might not be as bad as you perceive them to be. Consider that after Charlie Brown fell to the ground, he was probably concentrating both on his pain and how unfair it was that Lucy swiped away the football. Instead, what Charlie Brown needs to realize is that pulling away the football is just what Lucy does. It's in her character. Everyone reading the comic strip realizes what Lucy will do if she is holding the football and Charlie Brown goes to kick it. Once Charlie Brown accepts who Lucy is and what she does, he can stop focusing on the fairness of the situation (which only makes him feel worse) and better prepare himself to deal with her in the future.

It is unnecessary to debate whether Lucy is good or bad or whether her actions are nice or mean. It doesn't change how she acts. Good, bad, nice, and mean are all just opinions. Focusing on circumstances as the cause of frustrations in life will only keep you upset indefinitely. What is important is understanding how situations and people interact with your own actions and emotions.

Once you ignore what is fair or cruel and concentrate on how you normally approach and react to the experiences in your life, you can better evaluate if a change in action is necessary. Simply focus on how you feel. Since a pattern is cause and effect, any change in your own routine behavior will typically lead to a different outcome. Just keep in mind that whether you decide to employ a new approach or simply walk away from an experience, self-respect must be the guiding intention behind any change in action.

Technique: Cataloging Your Patterns

Section off a few pages in your journal and title each page in this section "Patterns." On these pages, write down patterns about the world that you observe. For example, you may recognize that whenever you fall asleep on the couch, you wake up with a backache; or you may notice that one of your friends regularly break plans with you at the last minute. The patterns you identify and write in your journal only need to be a sentence or two, and they do not need to be about anything significant or even about you. All you are doing is documenting the effects of actions in the world. Some may be your own personal patterns; some may be the patterns of others, and some may be your interactions with others. Whatever you see happening consistently, identifying it as a part of this world will move you closer to acceptance of what has happened and preparation for what may happen.

Update these pages in your journal regularly and create new pattern pages if you run out of room.

Take notice of the Lucys and footballs in your life. What situations are you repeatedly engaging in that are causing you grief, and are you reacting similarly with each occurrence? What actions of yours lead up to your undesired experiences? No pattern is too insignificant. Write them all down. Every little bit helps when working to improve your life.

It is equally important to identify positive patterns in your life as it is to identify negative patterns that exist. Recognize those people in your life who are continuously exhibiting respect, concern, and support for your well-being; consider what you do that brings prosperity into your life, and take notice of the effect you have on others by documenting the compliments you receive for your behavior. Don't take the good things in life for granted. Most people cry over the bad and ignore the good when they should be reexamining the bad and appreciating the good.

Approaching Different Situations in the Same Way

While many of the personal patterns you identify will be specific, meaning you act one way in certain situations and experience the same consequences over and over, you may begin to notice common themes across your patterns. Essentially, you may realize that you are approaching different situations in the same way. For example, maybe you notice that you are routinely lazy, messy, or picky. Maybe you recognize personal trends of having an addictive personality, difficulty making decisions, or a hard time saying "no" to people regardless of the situation.

Many of us have never recognized the similarities in how we approach different areas of our lives because we tend to focus on the details that make each one of our experiences unique. However, the specific details of any situation are rarely important; it is what a situation represents to you that affects you. Look at the way you eat, handle relationships, or view your job. Do you see similarities in the way you approach different situations? Your approaches may be similar because they are rooted in the same perspectives.

Because your approaches to many different situations are often the same, making small changes can have a broad impact on the way you approach different aspects of your life. For example, if you exhibit patterns of having a difficult time committing to both projects and people, changing the way you approach one can impact the way you approach the other. A little goes a long way when it comes to affecting your patterns. And when you begin to break a pattern and create a new one, you affect all the areas of your life that are impacted by the same perspectives.

The reason you encounter the same type of experiences, the same type of problems resurface, and you repeatedly end up in the same type of relationships is not mere coincidence; it is due to how you are interacting with your surroundings. You may take the time to debate how to handle each situation in your life, but in the end, you probably address them all very similarly. Everything in your life is linked together because you are in control of everything you do. Your patterns are not specific to circumstances; they are specific to you.

Changing Patterns
When you identify patterns in your life, there are two visible components: cause and effect. However, there is a third piece of the puzzle that is very important to your life: how you feel. The effect of a cause typically affects how you feel. Did you catch what I just said? Actions lead to results and those results can cause you to feel good or bad. In fact, sometimes the results are your feelings. Understanding how you feel is crucial because you determine whether a pattern is positive or negative simply based on how the cause and effect make you feel.

While the technique on cataloging your patterns will give you insight into how the world works, how you integrate with this world is the purpose of having that insight. Therefore, in changing your patterns, you must consider how your actions play into patterns that cause you joy or hardship. For example, if you identified a pattern that someone in your life has been consistently unreliable, you must also identify how that unreliability makes you feel. If it doesn't bother you, no change in your life is necessary. However, if it causes you consistent aggravation, you must change your action of relying on that person to avoid the aggravation it causes you.

There are three components to the previous scenario: 1.) You rely on person, 2.) Person flakes, and 3.) You feel bad. There are three components, but you only have control over two of them: your actions and your feelings. You do not have control over results. Therefore, you must cut out the middleman and change your actions to change your feelings.

Technique: After the Fact

Take out a small piece of paper and a pen. You can even rip out a page from your journal for this project. On one side of the paper in the top-center, write the word "YES" in all capital letters and underlined. Then turn over the piece of paper and in the top-center, write "NO" underlined and capitalized. On the YES side of the paper, write down activities that make you feel good *after* their completion: things that are healthy, gratifying, or fun. Examples may include working on a particular project, spending time with loved ones, taking vitamins, getting up early, organizing your home, or riding your bike. To get a jump on this technique, use the "Patterns" section in your journal as a reference for positive patterns in your life.

Do not put anything on the YES side that you enjoy doing in the moment, but makes you feel bad afterwards. For example, socializing with certain people may be fun, but those people might also get you into trouble often; maybe it feels good to vent about what bothers you, but you end up feeling exhausted and more upset when you are done. These types of activities will go on the other side of the paper, on the NO side. Based on your own experiences, you must decide which enjoyable activities personally cause you to feel bad *after the fact*. You may be surprised at how many regular activities of yours contribute to you feeling bad.

In addition to putting down activities on the NO side that feel good only momentarily, it is also important to write down what you do that does not offer any emotional benefits. Personal activities that don't provide pleasure during or after the activities are over are typical when you are depressed because you often feel like giving up on yourself. You feel like your life is a tragedy and believe you might as well treat it like one. When you leave depression in the past, you will no longer think this way, but for now, write down on the <u>NO</u> side of the paper any activities that are making you feel worse after you have done them.

When you write down behavior that belongs on the <u>NO</u> side, write the word "No" in front of the actions. This is so that when you read over your <u>NO</u> list, you are increasingly influenced to avoid those activities. You are literally creating a reminder list of what past experiences have taught you to do or not to do.

<u>YES</u>	<u>NO</u>
Getting Up Early	No Doing Drugs
Eating Fruit	No Eating Unhealthy Food
Going for a Walk in the Park	No Complaining
Drinking Water	No Sleeping During the Day
Cleaning Up After Self	No Looking at Pornography
Exercising	No Worrying
Meditating	No Cutting Self
Reading a Book	No Lying
Making Donations to Charity	No Socializing with Bad People
Doing Deep Breathing	No Listening to the Radio

You may have noticed that on the illustrated <u>NO</u> list, I wrote, *"No Listening to the Radio."* This may seem odd, but pop culture songs are often about love, loss, or hope, which are all in abundance when struggling with depression. This is commonly why people feel that the radio has a knack for playing depressing songs when they are feeling blue. It's not that the music selection changed; it's that you changed.

These lists are personal. You make them and you use them. What affects some people one way may affect you differently. You must decide how you want to feel and which activities bring you closer to or draw you further away from that goal.

Once you have written on both sides of the paper, fold it up and put it in your pocket. Keep it with you at all times, and try to remember what it says. If you forget, however, you can reach in your pocket and check your list. It might be a good idea to make a copy of your list in your journal just in case you misplace the list in your pocket.

Now here comes the action part of this technique. When you feel the desire to do something on the NO list, don't just avoid doing it; instead, perform an action on the YES list. You have the motivation to do something. So use that energy to do something beneficial. For example, looking at the illustrated lists, if you felt like eating unhealthy food, which is on the NO list, you could instead drink a glass of water or exercise (activities listed on the YES list). Not doing anything when you have energy will make the thought of doing something negative linger, and you are more likely to fall into the trap of doing the negative activity.

Trust me; there will come times when you really want to hang out on the NO side, eating poorly, smoking, complaining, or whatever is on your personal list. This will happen for two reasons. The first is because with depression, you stop caring about your own well-being. The second reason is the desire for instant gratification. It becomes nearly impossible to see beyond the temporary pleasure that comes from temptations on the NO list to their negative consequences, causing you to disregard the future harm you may cause yourself. There is a reason you put those activities on the NO side of the paper. *You* wrote them there because those activities have repeatedly ended badly for you. It takes discipline to break your patterns, and at some point, you decided that you would be better off not doing what you wrote on your NO list and doing more of what you wrote on your YES list. Your NO list is a list of warnings while your YES list is a path to fulfillment that you discovered by examining your own life.

Breaking your patterns sometimes means going against what you want to do. If you sleep poorly when you eat before bed, you may have to endure hunger pains before going to sleep. If you love your spouse but are subjected to his/her abuse, you may need to leave in order to end the assaults. The negative patterns that exist in your life are part of a routine way of living that is not working out in your favor. So going against them is supporting yourself even if it's not always easy.

If someone asks you for a favor or to do something, do not be impulsive in answering. If you are unsatisfied with your life, your impulses may be doing you harm. Tell that person you'd like a moment to think, or excuse yourself to the restroom so that you can examine your lists. If the requested activity is not on either list, consider on what side of the paper you believe the request or offer would be found.

If you believe the opportunity belongs on the NO list, turn the person down and do something on the YES list. Do not worry about offending others by attending to your lists. Your goal right now is improving yourself. And you will eventually find in life that the more you follow one side of the paper, the more you stay on that side.

Occasionally you may have an experience that you thought belonged on the YES list but left you consequently in a depressed state. Do not get down on yourself for the error in judgment. Remember, these are "after the fact" lists; and because of that, you won't always be able to tell which list an activity belongs on until you have had the experience. If you make a bad decision, note the experience in your journal and add it to your NO list if you believe that is where it belongs. There is no rush to discover all your patterns. You will notice them throughout your life, and you will make errors in judgment throughout your life. But as long as you are making an effort to know yourself, you will always be on the right path.

As time goes on, you will discover many actions that belong on one side of the paper or the other. Continue adding to your lists. Your lists will become longer and more accurate.

So keep a pen with you and update your lists with new actions as you learn about yourself. As the lists grow, so will you. And in time, you may find that you can safely remove certain activities off your <u>NO</u> list because you finally broke free from their control over you.

The more you learn about your interactions with this world, the more you will be able to integrate that knowledge into your life. Making change in your life is a big step, but consider that doing an action repeatedly creates familiarity, which is a feeling of normality. Just as many of your actions have become patterns through repetition, by consciously repeating new behavior, you can create positive subconscious patterns that replace existing negative ones.

Changing the way you typically act will require effort because you are used to doing something different. While changing your routine may require a few occasions of forced activity to get you into a rhythm, your commitment will turn that behavioral change into a new lifestyle. Humans have an incredible ability to adapt. Many people even believe that it takes just three weeks of consistent behavior to make or break a habit.[3] While some deep-seeded patterns may take longer to break, repetition will always breed familiarity. If you stick with the effort, you will be amazed at how quickly your life begins to improve. Keep this in mind as you put forth effort toward following the techniques in this guide.

The Feeling of Change

If you continue engaging in existing negative patterns, you will continue to feel bad. However, because you are used to those patterns, any change you make to your behavior may cause you to feel uncomfortable at times. This means that no matter what you do right now, there will be occasional feelings of discomfort at this stage in your life. This may make you question the point of changing your patterns. The reasoning is two-fold. The first point is that when changing your patterns, you will know that the cause of your discomfort is only due to the apprehension and work requirements of a new experience. The second point is that the discomfort you feel from acting differently will only be temporary as your new way of living ultimately become familiar.

The more you live a certain way, the more you solidify a pattern. The moment you intentionally act in a different way than you regularly have in the past, you immediately begin breaking a pattern and creating a new one. It will be your choice from that point whether to continue on the path of reinforcing the new pattern or to return to your long-standing habits. And while going against the way you have lived in the past may sometimes feel odd, it's probably just because it's been a while since you supported yourself.

Your experiences are a matter of cause and effect. The role of the past is not to stifle your life but to be utilized as a guide for recognizing the likelihood of events repeating in the future. The past is not definitive and the future is not obscured. Both are constantly changing depending on how you approach them in the present. The past can change based on how intensely you let it affect your life now and the future can change based on how much self-examination you do now. By viewing time this way, you gain the control to change the lingering feelings of the past and the potential depression of the future.

In the scientific experiment of life, you're the independent variable: the one that must change to affect results.

Chapter 5

The Truth about Bad Focus

As you use your journal to document your own personal patterns and the patterns of those with whom you surround yourself, you will begin to recognize details about your approach to the world. The knowledge you gain by identifying patterns will allow you to realize the probability of certain outcomes and act accordingly to make your life better. And when you feel good about your life, you have more energy to continue improving it.

In Chapter 2, you learned several physical methods to increase your energy levels. The methods discussed in that chapter, however, are only part of the steps necessary to increase your energy and motivation. As you begin to learn about yourself and the world, it's time to address the other way you increase your energy: by focusing your mental energy appropriately. I use the word "focus" because that is exactly how mental energy is gained or lost: by how and where you focus you attention. You might be excited about a vacation, restless because of an upcoming exam, inspired by a speech, or exhausted from an argument. And so as you focus on those things, your effort sustains your thoughts about them and consequently sustains the feelings they give you.

When you focus on something, you invest yourself into it. The return on investment that you get is an intensification of the way you already feel about what you are focusing. For example, if you are sad about a break-up and focus on the person who is gone, your sadness will intensify. If you are worried about a project, you will become more worried the more you focus on it.

Since most of us consider our own beliefs to be valid, we look for examples to confirm our beliefs about situations. Have you ever heard someone tell you that "you hear what you want to hear"? There is a lot of truth to this. If you are mad at someone, you will only acknowledge the bad. If you have a crush on someone, you will just see the good in that person. And when you experience depression, you look for examples of the world working against you. Think about those days when everything seems to go wrong. Does everything really go wrong or do you only focus on the negative? My guess is that plenty goes right on days like those, but by concentrating on what goes wrong, you only see the bad, making it seem as though *everything* went wrong.

This perception is what causes you to intensify the feeling what you are focusing on gives you. By focusing on what makes you feel bad, you don't just end up feeling bad; you also find ways to justify that feeling, which causes the feeling to remain inside you. And the more you concentrate on what is making you feel bad, the more you will convince yourself how bad things really are. So depending on what you are focusing on in your own life, you just might be creating a world inside your head that is filled with negativity.

Focus does not just increase the prevalence of something purely according to your perspective though; your focus can genuinely increase the prevalence of something in your life. Consider the concept of focusing all your attention on becoming rich. If you read several books on how to get rich, tried many methods on how to get rich, and were constantly searching for ways to become rich, over time you would likely end up rich. It doesn't mean it wouldn't take a while to get there; it just means that if you keep trying, you increase your chances of success.

Some people believe the opposite that when you stop looking for things, they coincidentally appear. This concept is caused by perspective confusion. What happens is that both things you want and things you don't want come into your life all the time, whether you are searching or not. Focusing on things tends to bring them into your life quicker than if you did not focus on acquiring them. However, it feels like it takes longer for those aspirations to transpire because you note the time it took from the beginning of your search until fruition. When you are not concentrating on a particular goal and it comes into your life unexpectedly, you do not acknowledge any passage of time because there was no exertion of energy. Therefore, while some may think that not focusing on what they want will bring it into their lives, that is really just leaving the future up to chance.

Those who are depressed often maintain one of two types of focus: a lack or an abundance of focus. In evaluating yourself, if your thoughts, fears, complaints, wishes, and discussions reference many problems in your life, you have a lack of focus. Too often people see all their problems at once and come down on themselves for their lives being a mess.

In some cases, people may think they don't have any focus at all and are, therefore, lost. However, it can surprisingly be the opposite. It may be that they are putting all their focus on the cause of their depression. In your life, if nearly every thought, fear, hope, complaint, or conversation has hints of a single person or issue, you have an abundance of focus. You are focusing so much on something you may not have control over. This is now the time to start focusing on your own life, not for anyone else, not for anything else.

The reason people sometimes think they have a lack of focus when they actually have an abundance of focus is because they have both. By focusing exclusively on a single issue, people tend to ignore the importance of everything else in their lives. They have an abundance of focus on one aspect of their lives and a lack of focus on everything else. In these cases, it's important to address the abundance of focus because that is what is causing the lack of focus.

In an effort to better understand these two types of focus, I will first deal with abundances of focus. Keep in mind that whether you are focusing all your attention on a single issue or on too many issues, both of these concepts presented here are important to understand so that you don't swing from one side of the focus spectrum to the other.

Abundance of Focus

When you have an abundance of focus, you tend to concentrate overwhelmingly on a particular issue. Essentially, you have a one-track mind in which you can't seem to stop thinking about a certain experience or person. The danger with this type of focus is that if you put all your attention on what you want and it doesn't work out, you lose everything that matters to you. This is often the reason people lose something important to them and suddenly feel as though the world is crashing down around them. They lost that which captured all their focus, and since they weren't giving attention to anything else, losing that one thing felt like losing everything.

In order to avoid the trauma of a loss like this, you must diversify your focus. Essentially, this is the theory of not putting all your eggs in one basket. Open yourself up to appreciating all the wonderful things in your life you take for granted rather than concentrating on only one thing.

With an abundance of focus, you not only risk a feeling of losing everything if you lose the one thing you focus on, but you also risk losing everything else that you take for granted. Remember how I said that when you have an abundance of focus on one thing, you have a lack of focus on everything else? Well, just as focus brings things into your life, a lack of focus will remove them.

When you lose something because you disregarded it, only then do you often realize how valuable it was. In these situations, your focus suddenly gets redirected and you start trying to make up for lost time and chase your loss. You put an abundance of focus (which is your pattern) on what is gone. What didn't seem to matter before now holds all your attention while you again continue to ignore everything else you have in your life and risk losing even more. You are collecting and ignoring instead of appreciating and enhancing what you have in your life.

If you spend your life chasing what you want and disregarding what you have instead of accepting the way things are and appreciating what you have, this cycle will be endless. You will remain unsatisfied as you constantly search for something else and always regretful that you lost what you failed to appreciate. There is nothing wrong with putting forth effort to reclaim what you lost or achieve something new as long as you appreciate what you already have.

At this very moment, you may be taking wonderful aspects of your life for granted. If your life seems to exclusively center on something you want or something you despise, then you have forgotten the many beautiful things that exist in this world, letting a solitary issue control you. What you are focusing on is probably not as much a matter of life and death as you think. It is not completely good or bad. It has qualities of both. It is, therefore, essential that you redirect some of your focus away from what you are concentrating on to what you are forgetting about.

Abundances of focus may involve a concentration on something you want, something you hate, or someone you desperately want to please. The feeling you get from your focus might be sadness, anger, or hopefulness; but the result is the same: the disregard of everything else in your life (the disregard of your own life). You look outward in one direction instead of looking around at all you have and inward at the person who is giving up everything else for just one thing.

The reality is that if you are unable to look past any one issue to see anything good in the world, it's time to let go of what you are focusing on. You are putting a value on it that is far beyond what it is worth. If any one thing in life ever makes you forget about everything else, it's time to walk away from it because it is probably the biggest outside influence on your depression. Even if you have already physically lost what you are mentally holding on to, *nothing* in this world is worth giving up everything else.

What you need to apply to your life if you suffer from an abundance of focus is appreciation. The way to appreciate more of what you have in your life is by reducing how much attention you are giving your current focus. And the best way to do this is to reduce how much attention you are giving *everything* in your life. It may seem odd that reducing your focus on everything would enhance your appreciation for what you are disregarding, but because you have little focus on anything beyond a single interest, the reduction in focus only significantly affects what you are giving the majority of your attention to. By taking space from your primary focus, you free up energy to concentrate on everything good in your life that you are missing out on.

When you take time away from your regular activities, you learn what matters and what doesn't. You become more aware of all that exists in your life. You learn to invest your time and energy into what you truly care about and utilize what you have in the most beneficial ways possible. Once you start appreciating what you have, the things you lose, want, don't get, or are hurt by will not consume your focus with such intensity because you will already appreciate so much about the life you have.

Technique: Lenting

In Western Christian tradition, the forty days leading up to Easter are called Lent. Many people will use this period of time to give up an indulgence.[1] While this book does not take any particular stance on religion, the act of giving up something from your life can help you recognize how important or unimportant what you give up is to you.

Try not doing something the next time you are inclined. Just temporarily stop pursuing some of the activities you want to do, whether that means not calling someone, having a favorite meal, overthinking an issue, going to sleep when you are tired, or complaining. It's not necessary that you wipe things completely out of your life, but giving yourself some space from your desires can help you recognize how important they really are to you.

You don't need to do the opposite of what you want to do. Instead, simply take a break from your usual routine so that you can try living your life in different ways. For example, you wouldn't be mean to someone when you want to be nice. You might just think about someone else's needs than you would have otherwise.

———

When you change your typical behavior, you have new experiences and new feelings. Lenting allows you to take a step back from your typical tendencies to assess what you want and have in your life. You may recognize that much of what you believe you need is not truly essential to your happiness. You may also begin to realize the importance of some of the things you have taken for granted. This means that by not taking action on every urge you have, you learn the true value of things: which things have less value than you realized and which have more. Essentially, you learn what truly matters and what you can live without. It may be scary to let go of what is familiar in order to try new things, but temporarily giving up what you want will give you the opportunity to create your life through your actions, not your assets.

Lenting addresses the behavior that you don't catch and address in your journal. The purpose of lenting is not to take your focus off what really matters to you but to change your focus when what you see blocks you from seeing anything else. It is lenting that helps you reevaluate the significance of everything you have and want out of life.

Lenting also helps you learn self-control. It teaches you not to pursue every interest. Your inclination will likely be to act as you have in the past, pursuing the desires you crave and fostering existing patterns that may be working against your happiness. However, if you are able to withstand those cravings, in time you will forget about most of them. You will be breaking the pattern of how you ineffectively focus your energy.

Lack of Focus

A lack of focus exists when you spread your focus too thin. Those who have an endless number of thoughts at once about a mix of different circumstances typically have a lack of focus in their lives. When you lie down at night, your head should not be spinning with thoughts. You should be relaxed. Too many concerns running through your head suggest that you have too many influences in your life.

When you feel as though your plate is full with responsibilities, desires, and predicaments, you have a weight on your shoulders keeping you from enjoying life. You feel as though the issues you must deal with are taking away from your happiness. To address a lack of focus in your life, you must minimize and prioritize.

Eliminating the "needs" that you don't really need and prioritizing where to focus your attention can seem like a daunting task. Everything you want and take on likely has some value to you. The problem, however, is not how many issues you have to deal with; the problem is how you view issues in your life. With a lack of focus, you are likely assuming the responsibility to deal with nearly every unsettled situation you encounter. You probably take on many commitments that you don't truly care about and feel the need to manage many circumstances that have little to do with you.

We all feel pressure to have a certain type of life. We hear the words of family, friends, our instincts, and even advertisements pushing and pulling us in different directions toward the lives we are "supposed" to lead. But the pressure you feel only comes from you. Not every issue requires your attention. While you may want to take on every issue with passion and commitment, determining what is worth your attention makes life a lot less stressful. It's time to begin sorting out your life.

Technique: Three Boxes (Minimization)

Because we approach many aspects of our lives in the same way, as a means of practice for how you approach the world, you can make positive change to your lifestyle by sorting out which possessions in your home are truly benefiting you. Essentially, use your home life to impact the way you approach your outside life and consequently your whole life.

Get three big boxes and mark the first "Sell," mark the second "Donate," and mark the third "Trash." Now go through your home and take everything you haven't used in the last two years and put it in one of the three boxes. You will choose in which box each of your belongings should be placed by determining whether each item is worth a substantial amount of money for your living standard (Sell), could be enjoyed by someone else (Donate), or can be thrown away (Trash).

Put any clothes you don't wear in one of the boxes. Find any knickknacks that you don't love and put them into the boxes. Take anything that was given to you as a gift that is not bringing you joy and put it into a box. Find anything that no longer works or regularly causes you stress and put it in a box.

You have three days to finish this part of the project. Once you have finished, take the "Trash" box out to the curb. You will have the other two boxes in your home for two more weeks. This is your time period to sell everything you placed in the "Sell" box. Once that two-week period is up, the "Sell" box (with everything in it that you haven't yet sold) becomes your second "Donate" box. At that point, take the boxes immediately out of your home to donate them. Feel free to give the items to friends, family, or charity; but do it quickly. You have one week to donate everything in these boxes. If that week passes and you haven't donated your belongings, those two boxes become "Trash" boxes; and it's time to put them out on the curb. Put the dates on a calendar or even write them on the boxes themselves.

Letting go of belongings you have had for a long period of time can be a difficult process, but it is an important one. Like the items in your home that you no longer need, you have likewise been slowly accumulating patterns and commitments over time that have led to your depression. It's important to learn how to let go of things in your life; otherwise, you will continually feel overwhelmed. And while letting go may feel scary at times, it can also feel quite liberating. Minimizing the items in your home can be a valuable step in learning to eliminate attachments from your life that you likewise may not need.

Now is the time to get rid of everything that is unnecessarily cluttering your life and holding you back from living independently of meaningless attachments. You aren't defined by what you own. You were defined by what did to acquire what you own, and you are now defined by what you do with those things. If you're not using them, they are taking up valuable space in your life. It's important to know that your life is based on what you do, not what you have. Prove it to yourself by walking your "Trash" box(es) of stuff you don't need anymore out to the curb.

Discarding insignificant belongings helps you realize that you may be engaging in relationships and activities that are not benefiting you. Think about it; every stress you have in your life is related to an attachment of yours. Problems arise with cell phones, cars, organizations, customer service, home repair, and anything else in which you invest your energy. So the less you own and the less you take on, the less chance there is for problems to arise that cause you stress. Obviously, you aren't going to give up everything in your life, nor should you; but by minimizing, you can better eliminate everything from your life that you don't really need, be it possessions, activities, dilemmas, or even certain people.

When you encounter feelings of resistance to letting go of things you no longer need, ask yourself why you want to keep them. "Because I want to" is not a good enough reason. Think about why you feel compelled to keep those items in your life. Is it simply based on comfort? Are you holding on to the past? Are you saving them for a possible future event? You probably don't need those things you hide away or keep in storage for years on end. Use them or let them go.

Memories may come up throughout this minimization process because of the sentimental attachment you likely have to various items in your home. Still, if the items you find are not benefiting your life, it's time to let them go. At the end of each day you work on this project, describe your feelings about this process in your journal, reflecting on how you felt and why you felt that way. Avoid writing in your journal while still in the midst of minimizing or you may lose the energy to continue the project once you stop writing.

This process takes less than four weeks and will significantly improve your ability to concentrate. If you are overwhelmed in your everyday life, your home probably exhibits this through clutter. You only have so much space in your home for things without it seeming crowded and messy. Similarly, you only have so much room in your life for things before you feel like your life is a mess. Physically minimizing what you have in your home will help you learn how to minimize the amount of issues you have in your life because you are creating a pattern. Less is more when you have too much. Everything in your home and in your life should be for a beneficial purpose.

Technique: One for One (Prioritization)

That is minimizing, but there is a second part of the project, which involves prioritizing. Once you have removed the boxes from your home, you can no longer bring anything into your home without taking something out of your home. Every time you see something you want, you will be forced to decide what you want more: what is available to you or what you already possess.

This technique will stop you from allowing your home and eventually your life to become cluttered again. It will also help you decide what in life is genuinely important and really worth your attention. You see, a lack of focus is rarely the fault of not knowing how to handle the issues you are facing. Rather, it is typically the result of trying to take on too much and, therefore, not being able to dedicate enough attention to anything.

There is only so much room in your life; you can't have or do everything. With only so much time and energy to devote to what you have and want in your life, it is up to you to decide what is worth keeping around and what you can let go. Recognizing something's purpose gives you appreciation for what you have. Recognizing that something is not benefiting your life allows you to more easily rid yourself of what is cluttering your life. When you take the time to determine something's value, you are given all the information you need to prioritize what you have.

Some of what you have, you don't really need; and some of what you have, you take for granted. Each of the focus projects helps you to examine your life and make determinations about what matters to you. And that is one of the most important parts of this journey: getting to know yourself.

Understanding Focus as Energy

Some people have a narrow focus and some see everything as an issue that they must engage. These are the extremes of focus, and as you learn to focus on what truly matters to you, that is not enough. You must also make sure you are using your focus in respect to energy.

Beyond what is important to you are the feelings that you get from what you do and what you don't do. Everything you do or don't do gives you some feeling even if that feeling is barely noticeable. This is where your energy comes into play. Your energy and your feelings are related. When you feel good, you feel energized. When you feel bad, you feel depleted of energy and consequently unmotivated to put forth effort toward improving the way you feel.

As discussed at the beginning of the chapter, whatever you focus on, you bring more of it into your life. Therefore, it's important to bring more of the things that make you feel good into your life by focusing on them. That positive feeling you get from what you focus on may come in the form of appreciation, a reward, or some life experience; but whatever form it takes, it's only necessary that the feeling be present.

Your energy is your most important currency in life, not money, not time. Energy builds on energy, and the only way you can give and get energy is through your own effort. You must, therefore, work toward things that give energy back to you in the form of a good feeling.

Exchanging existing energy for new energy is a lot like breathing; you must expel stored energy and bring in new energy constantly. You can't survive on the same energy forever just as you can't survive on the same breath indefinitely. So as you breathe your energy in and out, make sure you are breathing out into an environment that will reciprocate fresh energy.

Seeking new positive energy for the energy you exert is not doing something for a result; it is acknowledging the importance of being able to appreciate and utilize whatever you get in life. Results are truly just steps because of what you do with them. And if you give of yourself and get nothing in return, you have nothing to build off of.

Getting energy for giving energy will not always be easy. For example, climbing a mountain may be difficult; but it can create an inspirational feeling of accomplishment. Volunteering may take up your weekend, but it might make you realize how good you have it. Going for a run may take motivation and dedication, but you may feel physically rewarded when you are done. Keep your eyes open to what exists because, even though you may not always get the type of fulfillment you want from your actions, there are opportunities to gain from many experiences.

Getting a good feeling from what you do will give you the energy to do something else. And it is that energy you use to pursue new experiences and move forward. The energy you receive for the things you do may be represented in a variety of ways, which you may have wanted or not expected; but the "after the fact" must be some rejuvenation of energy. Every day, you choose how to spend your energy; and depending on what you give it to, you find yourself filled with more energy or less.

For many who have depression, they tend to put forth energy toward things that take energy away from them. They focus on circumstances that upset them and put themselves in situations that continue to have negative effects on them. Even if something feels personally important, if time after time you are left without a good feeling and feel personally exhausted, you may just have to give up what matters to you.

When you put your energy into the things that repeatedly stress you out, you bring more problems into your life. Some situations you encounter do not work well for you, and it's up to you to determine how much more time or energy you are going to dedicate to something that isn't returning you enough benefit. Sometimes, however, the reason you get stressed out over experiences is because you are focusing on the negative.

Negative things tend to have more weight to them than those that are positive because people see unfavorable circumstances as a threat to their happiness. So they focus on what is wrong with situations instead of what is right. They fight against what they don't want instead of going after what they do want. They have opinions that they are seeking to confirm rather than forming opinions based on what they observe.

Now I'm not going to try to convince you to strictly look on the bright side of life. Some things in your life may be causing you harm, and you'd be better served leaving them behind you. However, before you can make that decision, it's essential that you acknowledge what actually exists.

Everything in this world has good and bad points to it. What you appreciate is not flawless and what you despise has redeeming qualities. So the best way to know whether what upsets you is the result of a bad relationship or a bad perspective is to ask yourself if you can identify both pros and cons of it. If your opinion is entirely positive or negative, your perspective is likely skewed. Only when you can see the good and bad points of something, can you make a rational decision about whether to remove it from your life. Otherwise, you might let it go and then find yourself living with regret; or you might hold on to it and find yourself continually frustrated.

Technique: The Good and the Bad within the Bad and the Good

Take a moment to consider what you have in your life—physically, emotionally, and spiritually. Examine the good and bad aspects of what you have, no matter how insignificant those qualities may be.

You will probably have a very difficult time naming the good aspects of anything you loathe or the bad aspects of what you love, but simply realize that you're the one determining whether something is good or bad. So think about the friends, enemies, experiences, events, and activities in your life purely as they are.

Once you've done this pondering, open up your journal and create three columns titled "Item," "Pro," and "Con." In the "Item" column, write down three people, events, or experiences that you appreciate. Next to each item, write down one pro and one con to having the item in your life. Consider how the item is positive (pleasures, lessons learned, etc.) and how it is negative (undesirable consequences, loss, etc.).

Item	Pro	Con
Ex-girlfriend	Always says hello to me	Lies to me repeatedly
My cell phone carrier	Good reception	Bad customer service
Staying late at work	Possible promotion	Less time to spend with kids

Once you have filled in the pro and con columns for the three items you appreciate, write down in the "Item" column three people, events, or experiences that bother you. Write a pro and con for each of these items just like you did for the three items you value. While there may be more good than bad in what you appreciate and more bad than good in what you don't like, by only writing one pro and one con for each item, you begin to bring more balance into your life. You decrease the intensity of your love or disgust of certain things, enabling you to avoid getting hung up on them.

———

While everything in life has pros and cons, this doesn't mean you need to weigh every decision in your life with cautious scrutiny. It simply means that everything that seems good will involve some difficulty and what seems stressful always comes with opportunity.

When you are able to see good and bad in all things, you begin to have new perspectives because you see the other side of them. While right now you may think certain things in this world are either strictly good or bad, realizing that there is more to them than what you are seeing opens your life up to unrealized possibilities, including the possibility that what you perceive as bad might not actually be so bad. It will be your effort to learn about your relationship to this world that provides you insight into the benefits and drawbacks of your actions and experiences. And when you can look at the world rationally, you can make rational decisions about what's best for you.

The Call of Pain

Your focus can be drawn in many directions, but the place it probably takes you most often is toward your pain. I mentioned in the first chapter that pain resonates and exists for the purpose of signaling your attention when your mind and body interpret that something is wrong with you that needs help. The problem with this, however, is that by focusing on your pain, you end up intensifying the feeling it gives you. And for those who suffer from depression, this means an almost constant intensification of pain. You gradually hurt more and more as the pain eventually becomes overwhelming.

Whatever the pain may be fueled by, your control lies only in what you do with yourself. Some people will try to control the pain they feel by overriding existing pain with new pain. They look at situations outside themselves as reasons for why they feel bad and create new localized pain to divert their focus to something they are in control of. A primary example of this is cutting. Many people who experience depression cut themselves in order to replace existing pain that seems out of their control with new pain that they can start and stop whenever they want.

While pain calls your attention, more significant pain takes your focus off of less significant pain. And what often makes pain more significant is its timing. New pain tends to silence old pain because you focus on an experience versus a memory. By cutting yourself, you use the experience of physical pain to mute the thoughts about a life that feels bad. The problem is that while cutting may give you power over your pain, it doesn't change the fact that you are still in pain.

The reality of self-inflicted pain, be it physical or emotional, is that it is not a long-term solution to the pain you mute with it. Since creating new pain for yourself diverts your attention from existing pain, you don't end up dealing with a life that is calling for your attention. The new pain simply becomes a distraction. It really just prolongs the time until you take control of your life. But whether you try to control the pain by harming yourself or harming someone who hurt you, taking control of your pain is not in the ability to be the inflictor but in the ability to be the healer. Only by focusing on healing your pain do you increase the feeling of healing.

There are two basic types of pain: emotional pain and physical pain. In Chapter 2, we discussed several ways in which you can affect the way you feel emotionally by how you treat yourself physically. However, equally as powerful is your ability to affect the way you feel physically by how you treat yourself emotionally.

When it comes to the importance of focusing on your healing over your pain, the following technique may quite possibly be one of the most effective ways to overcome struggle when you feel mentally or physically beaten down. Because of the strong connection between the body and the mind, some people are able to alter their emotional state through physical activity and overcome physical pain through the focus of their minds. This is much simpler than you may realize and can be a great tool to help you through difficult times.

Technique: Reversing Roles

Focusing on your pain intensifies your pain. So it's important to understand how you hurt more: physically or emotionally. Sometimes this will be obvious. Other times, it will be difficult to tell. If you are having a hard time determining whether your body or mind is in more pain, try to determine which one was hurt first. Then you will likely know which aspect of your being is affecting the other. The next step is to heal the less affected of the two (or the one affected by the other).

Let's say that you determined you were emotionally distraught, and because of that, you also felt physically weak. Your mind is at the root of your pain. So instead of focusing on your emotional pain, you will need to pay attention to your body in an effort to give your body what it needs to feel better. You might go for a run, take a shower, or give yourself a massage. It's easier to heal your body than your mind because you weren't physically weak from physical stress; it was just a consequence of emotional pain. Trying to focus on making yourself feel better emotionally can often be too difficult when your focus intensifies a feeling.

On the other hand, if the pain you are predominantly focusing on is physical in that you are physically exhausted, sore, or sick, you need to concentrate on your thinking patterns. Rather than trying to use a weak body to fix your physical pain, take the opportunity to focus on what makes you feel good emotionally. This may mean catching up with friends, planning out a project, or watching a silly movie. The more you concentrate on what you appreciate, the less your focus will be drawn to your aching body and the less that suffering will affect your life.

Go easy on yourself by giving healing attention to the aspects of your being that aren't suffering as much. You may think this is avoiding dealing with the source of your problem, but healing any part of yourself is still healing yourself. And when it comes to living well, it's up to you to make the most of who you are.

While this technique can be very effective in improving how you feel, do not let it get in the way of your personal exploration of yourself. Just as feeling good can give you energy to improve your life, feeling bad provides the benefit of reminding you that there is still work to be done on yourself. But whether you feel good or feel bad, your continuing dedication to learn about yourself and your relationship with your surroundings will always provide you the opportunity for self-improvement and the positive energy you seek.

Too often we focus on defending our happiness instead of enjoying it. But when we fight for our happiness, we've already sacrificed it. You cannot preserve the happiness you have, which is why it so often feels fleeting. You remain happy by consistently putting your focus and effort toward what makes you feel good.

Don't focus on what you didn't get. Don't focus on the things that consistently stress you out. Don't focus on anything that is insignificant. And for heaven's sake, don't focus on the time you may have already wasted by focusing on those things. Focusing on what is wrong will only bring more negativity into your life. Some may suggest that focusing your energy on problems is how to deal with them, but it is focusing on solutions that eases dilemmas. All focusing on something does is increase the prevalence of it in your life, be it good or bad. When you concentrate on a problem, you typically become more frustrated. When you think about how to make the most of the situations you encounter, you do just that.

Every healthy relationship, be it with another person, a job, or an activity should always provide you with something positive in return. This is not selfish. It is the understanding that when you give of yourself and don't receive any benefit, you have a hole where energy once existed. When that energy is missing, you feel empty—the same feeling you have when you are depressed.

Even at its literal meaning, a depression is an indentation without anything filling it. And when it comes to your life, only one thing can fill your depression in order for it to disappear: energy. Take the time to examine the feelings you get from the different things you do. Take the time to recognize whether you are taking on too much or disregarding so much. This is your life we're talking about, and in a world in which what you focus on brings more of it into your life, you decide where to invest yourself.

*If you don't appreciate anything you have,
nothing will ever be enough.*

Chapter Break

Your Opportunity to Be Happy

Before proceeding, I want to have a heart-to-heart with you. You have an incredible opportunity in your grasp. This is your shot at life, and though at times you may think you have screwed it all up, I promise you there is time to change. Don't feel like you must force yourself to change though. See it as your chance to take the next step in your life.

While you have certainly made mistakes at times, that's one way you learn. Learning the wrong way can give you insight into what is the right way. Few of us get it right the first time around. I certainly didn't. But your past only follows you as long as you focus on it. When you make the most of who you are in the present, you take the next step.

Right now, you should own a journal that you have written in, have Yes/No "After the Fact" lists in your pocket, a pen to update them, a bottle of water at your side, been outside for fresh air and sun recently, and be sober. I'll bet you that last sentence does not fully characterize you. If it does, I truly applaud you. If it doesn't, take a moment and consider why you are reading this book.

What you have in front of you right now is opportunity. What you have inside you is potential. While it is true that you are the one who must get yourself through this life, there is more to this journey than just overcoming hardship; it's also about taking care of yourself. And when you have depression, you haven't been doing that.

Part of growing up means taking care of yourself, but consider what those words really mean. "Taking care of yourself" does not just mean doing what you think you need to do for yourself; it means caring about yourself by giving yourself credit, understanding, acceptance, and support.

Look at the bottom of your foot. Take your shoes and socks off and look at the sole of one of your feet. I'm completely serious.

Now touch it. Run your finger around the skin and watch the wrinkles move against your touch.

You are fragile. You are delicate. You try to put up a tough front, but you're vulnerable to everything around you. You feel more intensely than you let on. Yet as fragile as you are, you are hard on yourself. You may believe that you should be doing different things with your life, that this world should somehow be better, or that your life is not the way it was meant to be. But the discouraging, condemning, and critical tone that you have likely used to convince yourself to change has done little other than beat you down to the point of exhaustion, to the point of depression.

That voice—the one you use to get yourself out of bed, away from all that brings you down, and moving toward the good things that make you heal—must be lightened up. This journey doesn't have to happen overnight, and you don't have to be perfect. But what you do have is an opportunity to do things that make you feel good, do things that make other people feel good, and be proud of who you are. I know it's hard when you feel like you've made so many mistakes, but maybe part of the reason you aren't where you want to be is because of how you've treated yourself.

It's time to forgive yourself.

Say out loud, "I'm sorry ___(fill in your name)___."
Keep going (out loud)…

"I forgive myself for any abuse I have done to myself. For anyone I have hurt or mistreated, I will make amends beginning here. And so I forgive myself. I will try to live each day for that day, and when things don't go my way, I will not complain. I have complained and learned that complaining gets you nowhere but in misery that things aren't perfect, but things will never be. Yet as long as I try to make things great, that effort will be rewarding enough to make life feel as close to perfect as it can be. Not succeeding is not a tragedy, but not trying is."

Take a moment to write in your journal.

When you have written in it, fill up your bottle with water and take a drink. It's time to get your act together. It's time to treat yourself with compassion, respect, and patience. It's time to start giving life your all. Don't think that you can. Know that you will.

Go on, say it…"I will."

*Only through perseverance may we face
the challenges of today so that we may stand tall tomorrow.*

Chapter 6

Know Thyself

On the southern slopes of Mount Parnassus in Delphi, Greece, the ruins of the Temple of Apollo remain. This temple, dating back to the 4th century B.C. and home to an oracle, once held the inscription: "Know Thyself."[1]

These two words together make up one of the most fundamental steps in your journey through life. Being genuine is essential to living well, and yet many people don't know who they are, only who they wish they were. But who you wish to be is not what makes you who you are. How you live your life is what makes you who you are. Still, knowing yourself is something deeper than just what you do; it's knowing what's behind your actions.

Typically we feel the way we feel, stand up for what we believe in, and react the way we think is appropriate at the time. But why? Often people will back up their positions with responses such as, "That is the way it should be." But the question remains: "Why should it be that way?" Justifications for opinions may be based on experiences, rules you were taught throughout childhood, or just internal feelings; but there is typically something deeper guiding not just a few opinions but your overall approach to life. Understanding why you interact with the world the way you do is what it means to know yourself, and it is a key step in determining if your actions are being guided by perspectives that you truly value.

I do not deny the importance of trusting your instincts, but I likewise do not deny the power of suggestion. Movies, music, and speeches often inspire us to feel one particular way. Sometimes they encourage us to question our own beliefs, making us want to live differently. But if how you feel and what you do is guided by what you believe, it is important to recognize how your beliefs affect your smooth or turbulent integration with the world around you.

We often get agitated about situations without any understanding as to why we are truly upset. While many of us may blame the circumstances we encounter for our feelings, it is rare that we recognize our own perspectives that are guiding our feelings about our experiences. To understand why you feel the way you do gives you the power to focus on what is important while eliminating the excuses that convince you that what you encounter is both unfortunate and unavoidable.

Technique: Questions

You are involved in everything you experience. So the best method to recognize the bigger picture of what is bothering you in any situation is to learn about yourself. Learning begins by asking questions. So ask yourself lots of questions, and you'll learn about your own life.

Take any feeling you have and ask yourself why you feel that way. Don't start with the big question of why you are depressed; instead, focus on situational problems you encounter.

Ask yourself questions, and then ask yourself follow-up questions about your answers. For example, let's say that you are upset because someone stole from you. You might ask yourself why you are upset. Your answer would probably be: "Because someone stole from me." You might then question why you are upset that someone stole from you. Your answer might be that you no longer have the money to buy something you want. You could then ask yourself why you want that item. This process goes on and on until eventually you come to a realization that the reason you are upset about being robbed has little to do with the robbery; it has to do with a perspective much deeper inside you that might require adjustment to be able to manage yourself in this imperfect and changing world. You may even discover that there are other ways to get what really matters to you.

Don't look to other people unrelated to the issue to answer your questions. This technique is not meant for others to give you advice on how to feel better; it is meant for you to figure out who you are and why you feel the way you do. Therefore, you must provide the questions *and* the answers yourself.

Ask and answer your questions out loud so you can really hear your questions and responses. Find a private space and ask yourself questions, such as why events transpired the way they did, why you acted certain ways, what you want to achieve, why you really want to be involved in something, or why you even care about the circumstances that are agitating you. Try a range of questions and answer them the best you can, asking follow-up questions about your answers. In all likelihood, your questions may trail off a bit from the issue. This is okay. See where it takes you. Don't worry about asking the wrong questions. As any good teacher will tell you, "There are no dumb questions." This is particularly true when it comes to your own life. The more you ask yourself about your experiences, the more opportunities you have to learn about them and yourself.

This process requires time. So don't get frustrated if you don't know all the answers right away. Any answers you come to are better than none. The more possibilities you explore as reasons for your feelings, the more you will discover about yourself, situations, and yourself in relation to those situations.

—

Asking questions is a central technique to therapy. Therapists do not simply ask their patients questions so that the therapists can learn about their patients; they do this so that those patients can learn about themselves. You see, many people never question themselves. When you face so many choices and experiences every day, you do not have the time to question your feelings about each one. You just feel the way you feel and act accordingly. But both those feelings and reactions are guided by general perspectives that you hold deep inside you.

Over time, asking questions will lead to personal understanding and comfort. However, when you don't know yourself, as is the case with almost everyone who is depressed, the process of facing yourself isn't always easy. Sometimes it might even feel downright scary, but it is necessary. It means asking yourself the tough questions that you may not want to contemplate. Questions like what you would do if someone you love wasn't in your life, why you are doing what you're doing, and why certain things matter to you may require you to consider possibilities you never imagined.

Knowing the World around You

Just as you learn about yourself by answering your own questions, you learn about other people by asking them questions. While it's illogical to ask people questions about your own perspectives, if they are involved in situations with you, it may help you to understand their perspectives. Don't seek advice. Instead, question those involved in situations with you why they acted in specific ways and why they believe the perspectives they do. Very often we have a hard time accepting things the way they are because we don't truly understand why they occurred.

You do not have all the answers in the world, and your beliefs as to why people act the way they do at times may be wrong. You will have bad relationships if you always presume you know others' intentions purely by what you witness. When you ask others questions, you may even begin to question your own beliefs. Never stop learning about yourself and those around you.

Take the answers you get from others and ponder on them in privacy, asking yourself new questions based on their responses. The reason to ask yourself questions based on the answers you get from others is because *your* perspectives come from within *you*. What someone else tells you may ease your confusion, comfort your feelings, or make you upset; but there is a deeper issue that exists. Because you felt the need to question someone else means you were depending on that person's answers to determine how you should feel. Take private time following your questioning of another to question yourself as to why you might have felt certain ways based on the possible responses you could have gotten from that person as well as why you feel the way you do based on the response you did get from that person. It is an opportunity to learn about yourself and why you might be feeling or reacting the way you are in response to various stimuli.

Keep in mind that asking people questions may not always provide you with sufficient answers as many people act from their gut without doing their own self-exploration. They may not have questioned themselves as to why they acted and felt the way they did and, therefore, not have answers to give you. Or they may just not want to share their perspectives with you. In some cases, you may not even be able to ask questions of other people. Regardless, your exploration of yourself is not dependent on your understanding of others. Your knowledge of who you are comes from questioning yourself and understanding how and why you feel the way you do about the world around you.

Many people think they know themselves and the world around them well. They experience feelings and immediately believe they know why they feel the way they do. For some, their reasoning is to credit themselves for situations that make them feel good and to fault others for situations that make them feel bad. For these people, there is little growth in their lives because they are stubborn in their interpretations of their experiences.

There are also many people who simply don't know what's wrong. They spend their lives acting and reacting without giving the real reasons for their feelings much conscious thought. They only know that they feel the way they feel. Feelings, however, exist for reasons. They are signs that provide insight into the way you and the world are interacting, and it is up to you to explore your relationship to situations to understand your feelings about them.

Running from Yourself

Depression is an opportunity to break down your being. It emphasizes the importance of getting to know yourself, recognizing how your actions affect your feelings and vice versa. You are not dependent on the world to tell you how to feel. You are dependent on the world to explore yourself in various situations, yet many people use the world only as a distraction from facing themselves. You may just be spending too much time focusing on how others are acting inappropriately or treating you rather than understanding why you are feeling a particular way and what you are doing about it.

In silence, you are left only with yourself, which is why so many people use distractions to avoid facing themselves. They are scared of what they might find; however, facing yourself is an important part of overcoming depression. It is an important part of being the best you can be. Once you understand the reasoning behind your feelings and your circumstances, it becomes easier to accept yourself and take action to improve your life.

Too many people run away from their problems only to discover them again in new places and times. They believe that by moving, changing who they spend their time with, or making other environmental changes to their lives that things will suddenly get better. Many situational changes can improve your circumstances, but most of the time, it's not your surroundings causing repetitive problems; it's your way of living.

Until you take the time to understand your perspectives that are guiding your approach to life, you will continue to encounter the same experiences and feelings. While things don't always happen for a reason, they always happen because of a reason. And when it comes to your life, it's up to your inquisitiveness and acceptance to provide yourself the insight and confidence you need to improve your relationships with yourself and with the world around you.

The biblical story of Jonah and the Whale is about trying to escape God, but its underlying lesson is that you cannot run from your problems. You must face them head on. You cannot run from who you are. You must face yourself, understand yourself, and treat yourself with respect by living a life that makes you proud to be you. You have a great deal of control over your life, and that means no matter where you go, your life is not far behind. Your actions and responses will nearly always lead to the same type of problems if all you change is where you go.

You are not merely subject to the twists and turns of this world. You are the reason your life is the way it is. Your pleasures and problems do not exist around you; they exist because of you. This is not something to be ashamed of; it is something to be excited about because it means you have the ability to change your life at any point you choose.

Accepting Yourself

When most people feel any way but happy, they think of their lives as being different than they would like them to be. And many times these people respond by criticizing themselves for the way they feel. However, these criticisms rarely make them feel any better. In fact, these condemnations often make them feel worse because they don't just feel bad; they feel bad about feeling bad. They are essentially wagging a finger at themselves for living a life that they are already depressed about. So they feel both depressed *and* looked down on.

When you look down on yourself, it's easy to pile emotion on emotion. For example, when you are depressed and focus on that feeling with an eye to change it, what often happens is that you get depressed about being depressed. You make it more difficult to change the way you feel since the feeling becomes more intense the more you focus on it.

While you may not like everything you discover about yourself through your questioning, before you can make changes, there is a crucial step: acceptance. It may seem odd that you should accept yourself when you recognize areas about your life that you want to change, but it's essential that you accept yourself as flawed. You will have character flaws throughout your life, and if you won't accept yourself with flaws now, you won't accept yourself after you make changes to your character. You will think that you try and try to improve your life only to fail and fail. You might even feel that way now.

Many people refuse to accept themselves as they are, believing that only once they change will they be happy with themselves. But if you skip the acceptance part of making changes to yourself, you won't know which areas of your life need change and which don't. You will give up entire aspects of who you are, including strengths that you could use to overcome weaknesses. You will jump from one extreme way of living to another, and when you see any bad aspects of your new lifestyle, you will feel as though no matter what you do, you always fail as a person. But your failure is not your inability to change; it is your inability to recognize who you are and not come down on yourself for it.

Technique: Admitting Your Acceptance

Take everything you discovered about yourself through your questioning, and admit it out loud. Admit both your weaknesses and your strengths. Admit how you've screwed up and how you've overcome mistakes of the past. Admit what you realize about yourself; admit how you feel about it, and admit what you want to do about it. Do this in a private space, possibly one with a mirror; and meet the person you are. Admitting who you are is not always an easy process, and it can help to do it away from others. But truthfully, you're the only one who really needs to hear it anyway.

You may not have always treated yourself well in the past, but the least you can do now is be honest with yourself. By admitting truths about yourself out loud, you stop hiding from yourself. You put the truth out in the open so that all you can do is accept it. There isn't any other option. And admitting even those things you wish weren't true about yourself creates a sense of confidence in yourself because you put shame aside to be genuine.

You have a very important relationship with yourself that you have likely neglected for some time, and you owe it to yourself to develop that relationship if you are to be happy. By looking beyond the situational aspects of what is occurring in your life and exploring why you hold the perspectives you do, you discover whether those perspectives are working for or against your happiness. By then accepting yourself, you acknowledge what needs improvement rather than rejecting all of who you are.

You may not like who you are; you may not like the things you've done, and you may not like where it appears you're going. But avoiding facing yourself or coming down on yourself for who you are only puts you at war with yourself. And when you fight yourself, winning still means losing.

Improving Yourself

Knowing yourself and accepting yourself are not enough in this life. The point of getting to know who you are and embracing yourself, flaws and all, is so that you can take the next step toward improving the way you live. If you just learn about and accept yourself, you could end up feeling bad about who you are. You might simply accept that you don't have the life you want. But accepting yourself doesn't just mean accepting that you need improvement; it also means accepting that you are capable of making improvement. And the next step from there is making the effort.

Don't think so much about wanting to change yourself; think about wanting to improve yourself. Remember, what you focus on is what you bring into your life. The idea of changing who you are can sometimes feel overwhelming and make it seem as though you've wasted your life. Deciding that you want to change your life can make you want to take everything you have and have done, including many good things, and throw it all out the window, starting over from scratch. But there's no reason to do that, nor should you.

When you go to make changes in your life, build on the foundation of your strengths, of which I promise you have many. It's essential that you give yourself credit for the good points you have so that you can improve upon the lesser points you have. We all have areas of our lives that need improvement, and we always will. But it's the continued effort that we put forth toward improving our lives that keeps us continuously moving in a positive direction. And it's the acceptance of ourselves that allows us to appreciate the improvements we make.

You have a great opportunity before you. In fact, you always do. The idea of having a better life is what brought you to this book, and that desire must continue regardless of this book. You have it in you to have any life you want simply by living that way. But you can only work with what exists. Take the time to get to know yourself, be open with yourself, and make the choice of whether to do something about your life.

Your relationships with yourself and with this world depend on your commitment to each. If you are willing to put forth the effort, improvements will come. However, you may not always know what improvement looks like. So continue to learn about and accept what you encounter in others and yourself. When you are troubled, ask yourself why you feel the way you do. Learn about what influences your beliefs, your thoughts, and your feelings. Understand what kind of life those beliefs, thoughts, and feelings create. Then accept it all because that life is your own. That's what it means to be genuine.

Knowledge builds on acceptance and acceptance builds on knowledge. Each takes you a step further toward building your relationships with yourself and the world around you. As you develop these relationships, you open up the opportunity to improve the life that you have. And I promise that if you can do even a little bit each day to make your life better, it will be enough.

It's not the experiences that change your life
but the realizations you draw from them.

Chapter 7

The Burden of Choice

You spend every moment of your life experiencing your actions and the effects of what you do. You hear your voice when you express your happiness and when you complain. Your experiences hold lessons about the way you view the world, the consequences of your actions, and the consistency of your patterns. Your life is all around you, and it's your choice on how to live each moment.

At any moment you have a choice to make: to continue what you are doing or to do something different. Every choice is an opportunity, and you are constantly presented with them.

There are, however, few things in this world that you *need* to do. Thinking of your choices as "needs" makes them out to be something more than they are, but they are just decisions you make because they are what you want to do. It has been your choice to read this book just as it was mine to write it. At any moment, you can change what you are doing. No one is forcing you to live any way but you. Everything you do is your choice.

Choice, however, becomes a burden for many of us because we have been instilled with the "should." We are burdened by the idea of "should" from the way we think things should be to what we think we should be doing. Too many people avoid others because they believe those people are living a lifestyle contrary to how one *should* live. Others give up their dreams to do what they *should* be doing even though it makes them miserable day after day. Some people even hold grudges for years because another person didn't treat them the way they *should* have been treated. These "shoulds" take over our lives and distract us from pursuing what really matters to each of us, and so we end up unhappy.

Changing your perspectives or even reducing your stubbornness about them is hard because how your perspectives guide your behavior *are* your patterns. However, the likelihood that some of your deeply-held perspectives about what you should do contradict what's important to you is proof that you are not merely the result of others' beliefs. You may believe in something different from others, and it's okay to pursue that. Stop worrying about what others say you should do. Pursue what you believe is both important to you and makes you feel good. You are the one who has to live with yourself 24 hours a day.

Less Is More

Everything you do will lead to something else. While no one can know what doing in the short term will lead to in the long term, you can weigh the short-term benefits and disadvantages of your choices. However, saying "yes" to one opportunity almost always means saying "no" to another. Deciding to get up early in the morning, for example, provides you the opportunity to do more with your day; but it also gives up the opportunity to get more sleep. You simply can't have everything you want in life. Your decisions will take away certain pleasures and provide new ones just as they will ease difficulties and create new challenges. I can't tell you what they'll be. It's just the way it is.

The realization that your decision to embrace an opportunity is an abandonment of something else frequently leads to the fear of making choices. People become stricken with the fear that choosing means they will lose something from their lives. Ironically, people often fear losing things that don't even exist yet by saying "yes" or "no" to opportunities. They fear that a poor decision now could negatively alter their lives down the road and they may never encounter a similar opportunity again.

There are two factors that make a choice more difficult: its significance and the number of options. The significance you give to any choice is purely your own interpretation of what it could mean for your life. This is why it's important not to look at your choices as "needs" and not to put all your focus on results. Otherwise, the fear of making a bad decision can paralyze you with indecisiveness. And that lack of commitment to following through on any opportunity will repeatedly lead you back to the question: "What should I be doing with my life?"

In addition to the significance you might place on a choice, what makes a choice more difficult are more options. We tend to think that more options mean a better chance for finding the perfect opportunity. This, however, is precisely the problem. When you are left with countless options and you don't choose the perfect one, you get disappointed.

Here's the interesting thing: there is no perfect choice. No matter what you choose, you're going to be disappointed if you're seeking perfection. And because the choice is left in your hands, if you make a decision that leaves you disappointed, you blame yourself for choosing poorly. You then end up not just disappointed in your decision but disappointed in yourself.

We live in a world that offers choices to us constantly. Options often seem endless. And the less you know about what you want to do with your life, the more significance you will see in your decisions. People fear the vastness of opportunity and the looming need to fulfill their potential. This fear of choice that results from both one's perspective and the number of options leads to two typical outcomes.

The first common result from a personal fear of making the wrong decision is the seeking of advice. Lost without the willingness to determine the course of their own lives, people often turn to others for consultation. While communication can truly help gain new perspectives, people aren't usually looking for new ways to look at circumstances; they are looking to be told what to do.

People tend to seek advice because they believe others are better suited to make their own personal decisions. They doubt themselves and look to other people to make decisions for them. In this way, they also alleviate responsibility if they screw up because they have someone to blame for the poor choice.

Other people don't always know more than you, and they sure don't know what's best for you. No matter what suggestions anyone gives you, you have to decide for yourself what to do in each moment. Only you can determine what is really important to you and what you can live without.

The other typical consequence of fearing choice is endlessly debating what to do. Taking the time to consider your options is wise, but the point of debating is to make a decision; and the point of making a decision is to take action on it. By not making a decision, people tend to feel as though they haven't made the wrong choice. However, the longer you remain stagnant in your decision making, the more likely you are to lose what you currently have *and* the opportunity for what you could have.

While making a choice can seem scary, those who continuously mull over what to do without coming to a decision lead unsettled lives. They feel pressured and unsure about themselves. They don't trust themselves to make the right decisions, and so even when they do eventually decide what to do, they continue committing actions that counter their decisions like deciding to quit a job but continuing to take on long-term projects at work.

Choosing to do one thing while continuing to do another only leads to wobbling back and forth in your own life, never moving forward because of the fear of moving backward. But one choice isn't always worse than another. It is incredibly likely that you won't always see the ideal opportunity, take it, and have it work out seamlessly. More often, opportunities work out because you learn to appreciate what you are doing once you are doing it. So even if you don't make the "right" decision, what you do with that decision is more important than the decision itself.

When you make a decision, don't look back. Follow through. There are no long-term wrong decisions other than those that cause harm to people. Everything will provide happiness at some points and everything will create pain for you down the road. In those dark times, you might believe that you should have made different decisions. You might think that if you knew then what you know now, you would have chosen differently. However, if you always second-guess your decisions when you encounter difficulties, you will never be satisfied. You will perpetually be searching for a different choice to represent who you are.

You make your decisions with the evidence in front of you at the time with the knowledge of your past experiences in mind. And in each moment along the path that one opportunity led to, you are given another opportunity of how to proceed, just as you are right now. All that exists is this moment and all that matters is what you do with it.

The Choice of Who You Want to Be

The reason so many of us walk around with a constant dilemma in our path of what to do is because we are unsure of who we are. We typically just evaluate each choice and try to determine if it is what we want to do. However, since what we do both represents who we are and affects how we feel, choice can sometimes seem overwhelming.

So rather than putting all the weight on your choices of what to do to determine who you are, make the decision of who you want to be *first*. Let your intention of who you want to be guide your behavior. In this way, the choice of what you want is not so much outside yourself but of yourself. Your behavior ends up being both an expression and a representation of who you are.

Many people have never even thought about who they want to be. They typically just question the common possibilities posed to them. "Should I be a doctor or a lawyer? Should I go to school or get married? Should I travel or have children?" They look out at the endless possibilities for their future. They focus on the results of their lives rather than the effort it takes to get there. But if you don't even know the type of person you want to be, how will you know what to do with that life if you get it? Without knowing who you want to be, you won't have any real guidance on what to do.

If you don't have reasons for why you do the things you do, you lose sight of who you are. You could be anyone doing anything. However, if you know that you are an honest person, for example, you will commit to honest actions and know why you behave that way. It's essential that you understand why you make the decisions you make. Understanding *why* gives you control over your life. Your "why" (your reasons) are your principles.

Too much of your life, you have likely lived situationally, meaning you considered your principles based on the circumstances at hand. For example, you might have chosen to be honest in one situation but dishonest in another situation for whatever reason. This way of living only causes confusion. You need more stability in your life than basing your principles on your ever-changing present circumstances. You need to determine who you are and base your decisions on that instead.

Technique: Establishing Your Principles

To be able to make good choices, you must have good intentions behind those choices. When your intention is to honor your principles, your behavior always has meaning behind it that you value. In order to determine good principles for you to live by, consider what characteristics you value in others. Think about the people you admire in this world. What is it that they do that you admire in them? I'm not talking about what those people have or the repercussions of their actions, simply what those people do that you appreciate. Now think about what principles are represented by their actions.

Also, consider what behavior you appreciate in yourself and the principles that guide those actions. What are the principles that influence your positive patterns or the actions on the <u>YES</u> side of your "After the Fact" lists?

Beyond the principles you admire in others and appreciate in yourself, consider if there are any other principles that are important to you. Examples might include being generous, hardworking, fair, genuine, kind, or self-reliant. Think about the way you believe is the right way to live.

Now turn to an empty page in your journal and title the top of the page "My Principles." Then write down the principles you plan to live by. Write down what you believe at your core are important characteristics in an admirable human being. This is your chance to stop letting your emotions fluctuate solely on the changing experiences you have in this world. This is your chance to take control of how you respond to those experiences.

It's time to get off the emotional rollercoaster you have likely been riding and determine who you want to be. It's your choice whether to write in your journal at this moment, but if you think that dedication would be a good principle to live by, you might want to put this book down and write in your journal now.

Once you have identified the principles you plan to live by, honor those principles no matter the situation. When presented with an opportunity, a challenge, or a dilemma, act in the way someone of your principled character would act. Let yourself represent the decisions you make and the things you do rather than viewing yourself as a product of the decisions you make and how your actions are interpreted.

Not every situation will be easy or work out exactly as you like, but the ease or success of situations has little to do with your principles. What you get by honoring your principles is stability in your life. You gain confidence and pride in yourself. And that is the causal difference between whether you deal with depressing situations or depression.

You will surely encounter situations in which it seems that violating your principles would benefit you more than honoring them. You may believe that ignoring your principles is acceptable under certain circumstances. You may feel that one person's inconsiderate treatment of you warrants an equivalent response. You may even think that no one will notice you compromising your principles now and again or that a one-time exception is alright.

The problem with ignoring your principles, even on occasion, is that not paying attention to your principles makes you unprincipled. You end up scattered with your personality, unable to make decisions without second-guessing yourself, and uncertain about your actions. If one day you are honest and the next day you aren't, what kind of person are you? If you are usually trustworthy but occasionally break that trust, how can anyone rely on you? Actions do define you, but without you defining yourself first, those actions are inconsistent. It means that who you are is constantly changing. And how can you be happy when you are a victim of circumstance?

When you live by a set of principles, you always know what to do because there is meaning behind your choices. You eat a certain way, work a certain way, and speak to people a certain way when you know who you are. It is the principles that you live by that drive your personality.

Technique:
Incorporating Your Principles into Your Life

When you have been making choices throughout your life based on your surroundings rather than who you are on the inside, it can be difficult to suddenly give priority to a way of life that you are not yet accustomed to. Therefore, it can help to become familiar with your principles by reminding yourself of them on a daily basis.

Each day, look to your journal to read over your principles and then write one of them down on the back of your hand. This way, throughout the day, in good times and bad, you will be reminded of at least one principle that is important to you. If, for example, your daily principle is to be honest, avoid lying—even white lies or sarcasm. If you choose to be healthy, take care of yourself both physically and mentally. If you value learning, ask lots of questions and ponder on the answers.

Honoring your principles can sometimes be difficult. So take it slow. Do your best to represent all the principles you value in every way possible. You may only honor the principle you see on your hand that day a little more than had you not been reminded of it, but every little bit counts. Over time, your principles will begin to become second nature; and you will become someone you appreciate.

The process of honoring your principles truly depends on if you are willing to give up your dependency on results in exchange for a life without depression. Too many of the too few people who consider their principles don't live by them. They simply exhibit certain attributes to be viewed that way by others. For example, many people are not generous because it's important to them to be generous; they are generous purely because they want others to see them that way.

What commonly happens is that when those people don't receive recognition for their way of living, they lose sight of why they chose to live that way and consequently stop honoring their principles. The reality is that acting in a manner for others' approval is just living for results and puts your happiness and self-love in the hands of other people.

The absence of a defined intention of the type of person you want to be means that there is no clear thought preceding your actions. This leaves only the afterthought to determine whether you made a good or bad decision, making you completely dependent on results and others' opinions to determine your own opinion of yourself. In this way, you will never have self-confidence.

When you honor the principles you value for yourself, you don't just know who you are; you are proud of who you are. You stop becoming reliant on others to validate you because you know internally that the way you are living represents the person you want to be. Some people may not share your principles and criticize your approach to life, but your happiness comes from pursuing what you believe you should be doing, not what anyone else believes you should be doing.

Your principles are one of the few things in this world that cannot be taken away from you; they can only be given up. You see, in life, things will be taken away from you. People will die, items will break, and relationships will end; but who you are is not what you have, and it is certainly not what you don't have. Who you are is what you do, and when your choices originate with your principles, no one can ever take away who you are. You are in control of that. And you maintain control by remembering that which truly matters is not what others think of you but what you think of yourself.

We often view choice as a burden. We look at it as a defining moment in our lives that holds consequential significance and we, therefore, struggle with it. But you don't just have to make a decision; you get to make a decision. You get to choose what you do with your life.

Choice is an opportunity that only feels like a burden when you let it define you rather than you defining it. The struggle of circumstantial choice ends when you determine the type of person you want to be. This is the only choice you ever truly need to make in life. Every other choice is a subtopic of the principles you set out for yourself. Many of us get wrapped up in the details of choices, but the decisions you make are always the right ones when they honor the principles you value because no matter what happens, your behavior will always have meaningful intentions behind it.

Base your choices around the type of life you want to have rather than trying to determine your life based upon the choices you have.

Chapter 8

The Fight within Self-Esteem

Of all the things in this world in which to put your faith, what you should believe in most is yourself. Believe that you will honor your principles. Believe that you are making improvement. Believe that you can get through anything. When you believe in yourself, you are able to accept change within and outside yourself with grace because you know that you will be alright no matter what happens.

Now in all likelihood, when you encounter problems, you will be looking around to see who is supporting you. I have always believed that the irony of life is that our eyes face outward. I say this because it is so important throughout life, particularly in difficult times, that we look inward at ourselves and discover who we really are. Rather than looking for someone to blame or to depend on, look to yourself to overcome personal challenges. The reason I bring up this point is because when problems head your way, *and they will*, you'll see who your true friends are; but the one friend who should always be there for you is yourself.

During depression, you give up on yourself. You mourn your life. But how can you count on others to be there for you if you aren't there for yourself? Others can give advice, sympathy, or love; but unless you are willing to be your own best friend, their compassion will be meaningless. Your own lack of compassion for yourself will outweigh the support others give you. Your disbelief in your own capabilities will overshadow how much others believe in you. You will chalk up every good thing someone tells you about yourself as a lie or a fluke because you don't see what they see.

Let's be honest though; you do care about yourself. You wouldn't be reading and following this guidebook if you didn't. The problem is that while you want to be happy, you don't always believe in your ability to be happy. Supporting yourself, however, requires strength; and you are going to need it for the journey out of depression and the rest of your days.

You Hold the Light
The widely held belief that "you are the company you keep" implies that people reflect the attributes of those around them. While this phrase is commonly used to describe how people exhibit the characteristics of those they spend a considerable amount of time with, the similarities between you and another can happen in an instant.

Think about a situation in which someone is treating you poorly. You would probably feel pretty bad. In actuality, you are likely mirroring how the other person feels. Someone only treats another badly when that person feels bad him/herself. However, because of that person's treatment, both of you end up feeling upset. On the other hand, if someone is nice to you, you may feel good about that, in which case you are reflecting the positive feeling of the other person.

What you may fail to realize is that just as you are affected by others, they are also affected by you. For many people suffering from depression, they see the beauty in others but not in themselves. But those people shining around you do so in your presence *because of you*. Let me give you a metaphor to explain this further.

Imagine you are holding a flashlight with its base against the front of your chest. There is now a beam of light coming out of you and that light represents positive energy. Let's say it is shining on someone's face. From your perspective, the person's face is illuminated. However, since you are at the base of the flashlight, when you look down, you cannot see the beam coming from you. All you see is light on the other person. You, therefore, do not see yourself as having anything good to give to the world compared to the light of the person in view. So naturally, you don't believe others when they tell you of your greatness.

From the other person's perspective, however, he/she is nearly blinded by the light coming from you. The person knows that it is your positive energy that is affecting him/her. So the greatness that you see in the people around you may actually be, in part, caused by you projecting greatness.

You regularly project your own energy onto other people just by being yourself without saying or doing anything particularly meaningful. So sometimes the negative or positive energy you pick up on from others is actually a reflection of yourself. We affect those around us, and we are affected by the people we encounter. So take the time to recognize how you are acting and the general characteristics of the people around you. It will give you a good indication of who you are or who you will become.

When you look around at what you have in your life, you may feel lonely. You may feel unloved. You may feel like you can't do anything right. But you also have a much greater value than you likely give yourself credit. In fact, I promise that you have fans. That's right. There are people in this world who look up to you. You may not always appreciate yourself, but there are some people who are better off because of you.

The people who admire you are not always those who you want to like you, and those people also won't always exhibit their affection in any specific way toward you. Nonetheless, those people value you. If you're not sure what they appreciate about you, ask them. However, if you don't have the same appreciation for yourself, you probably won't believe them.

You very well may see a lot that is wrong with yourself, but there is also a lot that is right about you too. And until you begin to value yourself, you won't accept that anyone else truly values you either. How can you understand that others appreciate qualities about you if you don't see those same qualities in yourself? Without acceptance of who you are and appreciation for what you do, your mind will misinterpret how others view you. You will underestimate the value of others' kindness and overestimate the meaning of their disregard.

Perspective, Perseverance, and Appreciation

So often when we encounter negativity or hardship, we feel alone and at the mercy of this world. We feel confused, lost, and doubtful. And those times when we believe in ourselves the least are usually when we need to believe in ourselves the most.

Technique: Notes of Encouragement

The strength you need to pull through difficult times is inside you. It's in all of us, but sometimes we forget that. While you may spend much of your time lonely, insecure, or frustrated, you also likely go through occasional phases or experiences in which you feel good and believe in yourself. You will need to rely on those times when you do believe in yourself to pull through the times when you don't.

Take some sticky pad notes or small pieces of paper and write a message of encouragement to yourself on each of them. These messages should be personalized for you and your typical reactions to life. If you doubt yourself often, write something like, "I can do this," "I believe in me," or "This is my opportunity." If you get upset often, write something like, "Don't get angry," "Everything will be okay," or "Breathe." You might need to remind yourself to "Relax," "Smile," or "Be Disciplined." The words you write down may be your own or quotes that inspire or center you.

Now stick these notes in your home, office, or wherever you are likely to need to see them most. There is no specific number of notes you need. Maybe you need just one. Maybe you need several. Maybe you need some in different places where you spend your day. There is only one rule: your notes should not be lying on a desk or table somewhere; they should be taped on a wall so that they are at eyesight level. This way, when you need encouragement, you'll be able to rely on yourself to see exactly what you need.

As you get agitated at times during your day, look at the words you have written to yourself. They are words of you believing in yourself. They are reminders that whatever the circumstances, you are not in control of the world; but you are in control of your life.

———

When you are depressed, you have an eye for recognizing your flaws. You believe you're not as _____ as you should be. Somewhere down the line, you were convinced that you're not as talented, attractive, funny, experienced, or smart as you should be. And it is your beliefs about yourself that guide your approach to life. Remember how you chose principles to guide your everyday decision making? Well, when you are principled, all you are doing is viewing yourself a certain way and acting on that perception of yourself. By that same concept, if you see yourself as attractive, you will act with confidence about your looks and almost never doubt this belief. If you see yourself as unintelligent, you will interpret any difficulties trying to learn something new as personal failings rather than challenges that anyone learning must face.

Your perspectives have a significant impact on what you do and how you feel. The way you view yourself is the person you will become because you are both on the critiquing end and on the receiving end of those critiques. I am in no way encouraging you to convince yourself of a truth that doesn't exist. However, there is a big difference between accepting yourself the way you are and believing truths about yourself that are completely subjective. The way you view life is directly linked to the way you experience it.

Any negative thoughts about yourself can lead you to a depressed life because your focus will intensify your feelings about personal inadequacies, and that intensity can make those qualities seem overwhelming and nearly impossible to change. Therefore, either your actions need to change to affect your perspectives or your perspectives need to change to affect your actions. In either case, you affect your feelings.

It's natural to think that qualities like your physical appearance or intelligence are unchangeable and, therefore, no behavioral change will affect who you are. This is again why it is necessary to accept yourself. Once you accept who you are and become okay with that, you can then take control of your life. No one looks good all the time. No one is right all the time. But you dress yourself up or read a book. So many people grow up with the belief that they could be anyone or do anything with their lives, but when life knocks them down a few steps, they quit, believing that they were the reason. The truth is they were the reason *only* because they gave up.

There is a story that I recall about a young boy standing in a field with a baseball and a bat. He declared out loud "I am the greatest hitter in the world," tossed the ball up into the air, and swung to hit the ball as far as he could. He missed though, whizzing around in a circle and nearly falling over. So he picked up the ball, again said "I am the greatest hitter in the world," and tossed the ball up in the air. Again, he swung and missed. And then on that third try, he grabbed the ball and bat, said "I am the greatest hitter in the world," tossed the ball into the air, swung as hard as he could, and missed the ball. Whizzing around in a circle from his swing, he collapsed onto the ground, picked up the ball, and said "I am the greatest pitcher in the world."

This story is both about perspective and perseverance. Rather than think narrow-mindedly that being a good hitter was the only option, the boy saw that he had also tossed the ball in the air and struck out whom he considered to be the greatest hitter in the world, consequently making him the greatest pitcher in the world. There is always a different perspective to every experience. You get to decide which one you collapse on.

In any situation, you can focus on what is wrong with it or what is right with it; and whichever one you focus on will affect how you feel. You could see yourself taking a lonely walk or exploring the world. You could see yourself as unwilling to make a commitment or sampling life to discover what you like.

Too often many of us focus on the negative side of experiences. We see precisely what we want and any failure to get that seems like a complete failure. However, the more specific you view your success, the less open to success you will be. Looking outside the box is something that comes from putting forth effort. It's not just essential that you put forth effort into accomplishing a goal but that you put forth effort into believing in yourself. Whenever you find yourself pained, consider ways that the troubling situation might just benefit your life. When you are open to possibility, you are also open to opportunity.

Opportunity is everywhere, and it is up to you to pursue it if you choose. Because you are what you do, your talent to push through challenges lies in your perseverance. Your strength does not come from convincing yourself that you deserve something. It doesn't even come from doing what you're good at. It comes from doing what you think you're not good at. And the only way to be good at anything you're not good at is through practice. Struggle is not a sign of failure; it's a sign of growth. It's the process of learning to do things better. That's why you're reading this book. You've had difficulty being good at living, but you're not going to quit. You are learning how to do it better. That's what this is all about. It is your effort that always makes you who you are.

The problem with effort can come into play because of the credit you may fail to give yourself. I have known so many people, including myself, who put stumbling blocks in front of themselves to prove they could overcome challenges. What happens is that they either don't accomplish their goals and criticize themselves for their lack of ability *or* they do accomplish their goals and don't pat themselves on the back. They don't give credit where credit is due, making those stumbling blocks nothing more than added stress. The story about the boy tossing the ball to himself showed effort, but throughout the story was appreciation. Your effort gives you the power to do nearly anything in this world, but a lack of appreciation for that effort makes it all worthless.

Appreciation is what gives everything a purpose, which gives your life value. You can have everything you need (and you just may right now), but if you don't appreciate it, it does you no good. Instead of wanting what you can't have, use everything you do have to be the type of person you want to be.

If you constantly focus on wanting life to be different instead of making the most of the life you have, your focus will be on a life that doesn't exist. Since your focus intensifies what you are concentrating on, you will only become more aggravated about the life you want that isn't there.

What you don't have does not exist and, therefore, has no value. And if you don't appreciate what you have, you do not value that either. Therefore, if you are always seeking something you don't have and never appreciating what you do have, essentially nothing in your life has any value.

Often with depression, people aren't satisfied. They are frequently looking for more instead of appreciating what they are getting even if it's miniscule. They look at their lives and think they're not as good as they could be. But what you are searching for to fill the emptiness in your own life isn't *out* there; it's *in* you. Fulfillment comes not from acquiring or accomplishing something but from appreciating it. You can climb the tallest mountain to feel complete, but if you don't pat yourself on the back for what you've done, your effort will be in vain. Without appreciation for what you do, you'll always be searching for what will make you happy; but you'll never find it.

The way to enhance appreciation is to reduce your focus on your specific goals. Just like the boy whose specific goal was to hit the ball as far as he could, his ability to appreciate himself was not dependent on the outcome of his goal. He accepted what happened and found appreciation in his own ability to pitch (which wasn't even a goal for him). There are many ways in this world to find happiness, not just one particular path you may be set on taking.

Negativity

Self-esteem is more than simply how you view yourself; it is how you view your life. Both your feelings about yourself and those you have about your experiences are often similar because one seems to cause the other. And with depression, when you focus on what's wrong with yourself and you focus on what's wrong with the world, neither gives you a reason to feel good about the other.

During my time with depression, I was critical of people. I would judge them with an eye for imperfection while simultaneously demanding perfection from them (which, of course, I never got). I would find something wrong in everything. If I wasn't invited somewhere, I would feel left out. If I was included, I would feel burdened by not having enough time for everything. My interpretation of my surroundings was always negative, and consequently, I was never happy. How could I be when I focused on what was wrong in everything?

There wasn't anything in my life that was inherently bad. What was happening was that because I was depressed, I would look for the negativity in situations. I would subconsciously focus on what was wrong in situations to give me a reason for why I felt bad. It would confirm that I was right to feel bad because everything else was wrong, but despite this approach, I never ended up feeling better, only worse. I was simply blaming what was around me for the way I felt instead of taking it on myself to improve the way I felt.

When you find negativity in many areas of your life, learning to appreciate any aspects of a situation will allow you to leave the negativity behind you and move on without concentrating on your disappointment. To understand that good will always come your way over time, look back at anything you ever considered to be bad in your life and come up with reasons why it may have been for the best. Even if you believe that aspects of your life might be better off had a situation not gone as it did, think about any pleasures or opportunities that indirectly resulted from the negative experience that might not have transpired otherwise.

Technique: The Bad that Created the Good

Grab a pen and divide a page in your journal into two columns. Title the column on the left "Bad Experiences" and list hard times, regrets, and mistakes in your life. Then title the column on the right "Good Experiences" and write down everything good you appreciate about your life. Now draw a line connecting which bad experiences caused the good experiences in your life to take place, even if the role it played was slight or indirect. For example, perhaps if you hadn't lost a relationship with a lover, you might not have moved to a new city, in which case you would not have gotten a job where you met someone wonderful. Anything can lead to anything else over time, and without some of the experiences you hate, you won't get some of the experiences you love. You will begin to discover through this project and your own life experiences that no matter what happens, good times will eventually come to pass as a result.

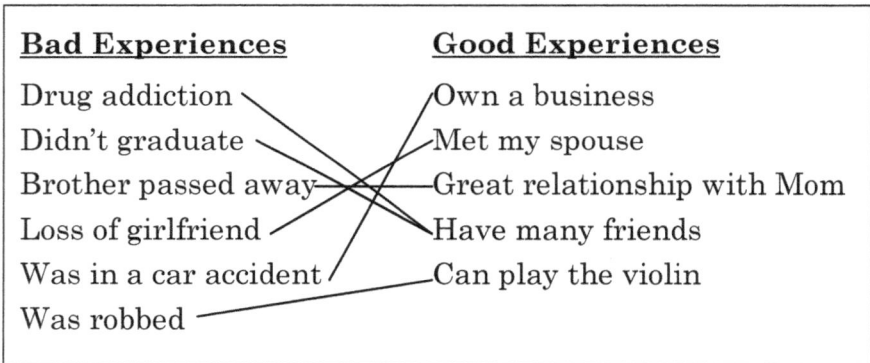

Bad Experiences	Good Experiences
Drug addiction	Own a business
Didn't graduate	Met my spouse
Brother passed away	Great relationship with Mom
Loss of girlfriend	Have many friends
Was in a car accident	Can play the violin
Was robbed	

You will not need to connect all the bad experiences on the left side of the page to all the good experiences on the right side of the page. Many of the bad experiences in your life have not yet brought about good that you can see. And you probably don't remember many of the bad experiences that led to the good aspects of your life because you let go of those negative experiences. However, try your best to recognize the connections because, believe me, they exist. As you continually update the left and right sides throughout your life, you may be surprised in the future (possibly even years from now) that some of what you write down now that is problematic will be connected to great experiences in your life down the road.

When you look at the illustrated technique, it may not make any sense to you. You might question how a car accident could lead to someone owning a business. The connections may not be clear to anyone other than the person who made the list because one thing might lead to another, which leads to another, and so on. Your journey from bad to good may be lengthy, but you always get there over time. During times of hardship, the distant future may be unknowable; but the long-term effects of difficulty will always have aspects of pleasure.

—

When you are stuck in a pattern of negativity, it's common to reject circumstances, believing they are nothing but trouble for your life. This technique, however, starts implanting the subconscious understanding that no matter what you do or what happens in this world, good times will eventually come to pass because of it. There are surely negative patterns you need to identify and address to avoid causing yourself problems and making the road to happiness longer than it needs to be. Still, over time good experiences will come into your life, some of which you might not appreciate as much if you hadn't gone through tough times to get there. Spring always comes no matter how cold, dark, and lonely winter seems.

Next time you encounter a frustrating situation, take a moment to question whether you can foresee anything good coming from it. You may not be able to think of anything at the time, but make the effort anyway. Look at the situation from all sides, open to the possibilities of what it could lead to, not just the bad that could come from it. It just might make the situation a little easier to handle. One day soon, when you have a bad day and someone asks you how your day was, you might just find yourself saying, as I did, "A lot of good happened today depending on how you look at it."

Doing the Right Thing

In order to eliminate negative feelings about this world and yourself in this world, you must go beyond changing the way you view the world inside your head. You must also change the way you treat the world outside your head by considering the welfare of others. This way, you will become a central player in making the world (that you may find to be so bad) a better place.

I've wrestled with this concept a lot. In depression, you focus almost exclusively on how you feel or don't feel. You don't really think of others' needs as worth your energy because your own suffering takes up most of your attention.

Now I've heard all my life people preach to me about helping others and leading a moral life. Never one to take what I hear at face value, I questioned why. They'd cite obligation, scripture, or experiences that they had. But what I saw in the news and around me were people hurting others, talking about others behind their back, stealing, and lying. In response, I saw no need to care for others who didn't care for me. I saw no need to live morally in a world where so few did. So I focused on me instead of them—what I wanted rather than what was ethical—and that turned out to be a huge mistake. It turned out that doing what was right in my treatment toward others had more overall personal benefits than ignoring morality for what seemed to benefit me in the moment. So why does doing what is right really matter?

It matters because a life of morality is directly proportional to happiness, and there are several reasons for this. The morals that affect your happiness are not those that address how you believe the world *should* be. They are not about defending a pro-choice or pro-life stance. They are not about supporting wars you believe are justified and protesting those you see as criminal. They are not about judging how others act. The morals I speak of are about core human principles, such as generosity, compassion, honesty, and respect—the morals that affect how you relate to people.

The first reason to do the right thing is to take control of your life. Criticizing the way things were never made anything better for me. In fact, it made things worse. But by doing something about the problems I saw, I gained control of my life. I was no longer a victim in a world of devastation; I became an active contributor in improving what I saw wrong in the world. If I didn't want to see cheats in the world, I couldn't be one.

There was a time when I thought that doing the right thing was actually a loss of control. It seemed that those who committed to being ethical would eventually experience someone taking advantage of them. I would witness these betrayals and feel like those people had been suckers for being upstanding individuals.

What I came to realize is that if you look at the inappropriate way some people act and use that as a reason to act unethically, then you are allowing others to tell you what to do by example. If you think you are nice but someone makes you angry, who is really in control? There will always be people who will take advantage of you, but there are many more who will appreciate your commitment to a code of ethics. Rather than letting a few bad apples tell you who you should be, be the type of person you wish there were more of in this world.

The second reason to do the right thing is because of the similarities in the way you approach different aspects of your life. When you show love, concern, and respect for others, you inadvertently show those same displays of affection toward yourself. And God knows you need that self-love. That's what this chapter is all about.

The third reason is that when you treat others well, many times they show their gratitude. This gives you a feeling of importance. It is likely that you feel you aren't doing anything substantial with your life. You may yearn to be someone great or for your life to have meaning. What more influential a role could you play in this world than bettering the lives of those whom you encounter? People need you just as you need them from the moment you first go outside each morning.

What I must tell you is that even though others' appreciation will make you feel good, you won't always get "thank yous," respect, or even an acknowledgement of your effort from them. While this might make you want to return to a life of not caring, thinking that you aren't making any difference, consider the life of a teacher. Teachers dedicate their lives to helping educate others, but they probably only have a substantial influence on one person in each class. That's a small ratio, but they stick to their effort because that one person in each class depends on them. Can you imagine if those teachers gave up? Similarly, you cannot give up when you don't get the type of responses you would like. Even if not everyone appreciates your ethical nature, some need it desperately. And believe me when I say that you are one of those people who desperately needs you to be ethical. You need to be someone whom you can believe in.

The fourth reason to do the right thing is because you are a witness to the way you live. You are the only one who always knows the intentions behind your actions, and by living ethically, you gain pride in yourself that you are a good person. You know that no matter what comes your way, you will do what is right. You become a first-hand witness to the actions of someone who is living an upstanding life. You are constantly around this person who stands up for the greater good, and then you realize that the person doing all this is you.

The only way to love yourself is to love the way you live. There are always opportunities and aggravations tempting you to give up your morality, if even for a moment when no one is looking. But you are always looking, and it's time that you set an example for yourself. The simple fact is that not living morally makes you a constant witness to immorality, and as a result, you will continuously come down on yourself for not living up to your potential.

There may be more reasons to do the right thing. These are just the ones that stood out to me. It turned out that being a good person was simply part of playing the role of the person I wanted to be. And so doing what was morally right made me appreciate the person I became.

When you do the right thing, be humble. There is no reason to shove your integrity in others' faces. People notice your actions even if they don't always give you recognition, and the point is not to set yourself apart from others or above them. The beneficial consequences of living morally do not come from others rewarding you; they come from you appreciating your own life.

When you see a world that is filled with problems, you may just want to give up, acting selfishly without regard to morality. And while you may not always see the beneficial effects of doing the right thing, the damaging effects of doing the wrong thing tend to stand out. You turn yourself into exactly what you despise in the world.

All the pain you feel, all the doubt, all the fear, and all the anger will not go away until you realize how great you are. But in order to see your greatness, you have to do things that make you a great person. Give to others, be kind, compliment people, show your respect, and live by the many other morals and principles that honor doing the right thing. The way to increase the intensity of your positive qualities is to increase the frequency of their use.

The Cost of Happiness

Happiness comes at a price. It means doing the right thing even when you might not want to abide by your morals. You will not be able to lie to avoid the consequences of misbehavior, and you may occasionally have to spend a few extra dollars to be honest and considerate. You won't be able to eavesdrop on conversations that could provide you important insight, and you won't be able to cheat just to get what you want. When you commit to doing the right thing, you will not get the advantages that come with ignoring morality; but you will gain pride in the way you have chosen to live your life. And when you are depressed, pride in yourself is more important than anything you could sacrifice it for.

You will feel badly over time if you live unethically, even if that behavior is infrequent. Feelings of guilt, fears of being judged, and disappointment in oneself are pervasive traits in someone who doesn't tend to morality. What would you rather feel: eased situations with persistent feelings of self-loathing (which you may have now) or challenging situations that you can learn from while simultaneously being happy at the life you live?

Before you answer that question, there is yet another cost of happiness to consider, which I briefly mentioned earlier. By being kind and generous, you will not only give up advantages here and there; you will also be taken advantage of on occasion. A small percentage of the time, people will take advantage of your generosity and kindness. Some will question your authenticity; some will try to discredit your good will, and some will encourage you to cave on your morals now and again. This may happen because those people do not care about their actions or they may just not care about yours. Whatever the reason, it will happen.

Consider these experiences tests of your willpower to maintain your moral nature. They may make you question the way you live, and there is nothing wrong with that as long as you recognize the value of your upstanding nature to yourself and to others. Every now and then, living well causes frustration; but by and large, it creates a life you appreciate.

So what is your answer? Is happiness worth the cost of happiness? Everyone I have ever asked who has paid the price of happiness believes it is worth it. Maybe you will too (because it is).

Not Everyone Will Like You

You should know that living a moral lifestyle makes you like who you are over time, but it does not always yield the friends you desire. In fact, no matter what you do in life, someone will always complain about your actions. While this might seem upsetting at first, the knowledge of this inevitability can actually be quite liberating. You begin to realize that one person complaining does not mean there is something wrong with what you are doing but that people complaining is just a part of life.

No one likes rejection. It feels bad to be excluded, looked down on, or singled out; but the opinion of a few is not always representative of the opinion of many. Those people who are satisfied rarely speak up, but those who are dissatisfied often do. News stories are typically about troubling situations. Talk shows tend to be filled with people whining. The voices that seem to stand out the most are usually not those complimenting you but those disagreeing with you. But whatever you hear, no one comment is ever the whole truth.

Acknowledging the discontent of those who complain about you is fine. They may have valid points that are worth listening to and applying to your life, but they are just perspectives. Their opinions may be purely selfish desires that are not the greater will of the people around you or even that of yourself. If you get stuck focusing on the complaints of the few and disregard the silent majority who may support you, you will ignore everything great you are creating. You will feel like you can't win. You will get stressed out, and in trying to please everyone, you will appear indecisive. Hence, the reason so many politicians seem to flip flop on their ideals.

In accepting that someone will always complain, you also begin to accept that not everyone will like you. This gives you incredible freedom as you stop living for other people and start living for yourself. Bill Cosby once said, "I don't know the key to success, but the key to failure is trying to please everybody."[1]

Trying to satisfy everyone's desires all the time will overcomplicate your life. You will delay making decisions only to be disappointed when someone complains about the choices you make. So often the reason situations seem complicated is because we take into account too many factors. In fact, nearly every time I have ever heard someone say that a situation was "complicated," the answer was really very simple. We are typically the ones who make situations feel complicated. In life, you will make decisions that others won't always like; but in the end, you are the one who has to be content with the way you live and the intentions guiding your actions.

When you stop trying to please everyone, you worry less about everything you do and everything you want to do. Some might believe that the fear of doing the wrong thing is what keeps them doing what's right. But for many people, that fear is really just holding them back. They focus so much on how they think they've screwed up that they stop thinking about how they can move forward. They worry so much about saying the wrong thing that they don't end up saying anything at all. They spend so much time living in fear that they don't even enjoy what they have while they have it.

One of the biggest advances I made in overcoming my own depression was when I gave up the need to be liked by others. I stopped being concerned with who said what and no longer interpreted others' behavior as a commentary on me. I focused more on what I believed was right than on how people viewed me, and soon all that began to matter was whether I liked myself.

Your view of yourself cannot be based on others because when you are alone, you have to be okay with who you are. Too often people live for those around them. They seek to please them without nearly as much consideration for themselves. They are constantly concerned about how others view them. They believe that whether others approve of their lifestyle is a determining factor in whether they are good or bad people. But you are well aware of what makes someone a good or bad person. You know what is appropriate and what is deceitful. It is in the attempt to consistently get a thumbs-up from those around you that you stop considering the opinion of the one who matters most: you.

Being overly concerned with whether people like you will intensify your depression. You will stop being nice because you enjoy being a nice person and start being nice specifically so that others like you. And anytime another is not overtly affectionate, you will think you are doing something wrong and become unnecessarily self-conscious.

Getting over depression will not come from others telling you that you are a great person. It will come from you believing it. When you live ethically and take pride in that, you are no longer dependent on others to tell you if you are doing what's right. You already know you are, and because of that, you have reasons why others would be proud of you too. There is always room for growth, but when you are proud of the life you live, you stop fearing that others are looking down on you. The time has come to stop depending on the inconsequential validation of others and make the conscious effort to, once and for all, honor a lifestyle that *you* believe makes you a good person.

Giving up the need to be liked by everyone does not mean you stop showing affection toward others. It just means that you stop depending on them to validate your self-esteem. When you concentrate your effort toward being the type of person you think others will like rather than just being yourself, you give up your greatest strength: being genuine. Hiding behind a veil because of how others might react to the real you is not living. Now is the time to start being yourself regardless of what those around you may think. By realizing that there will always be someone who doesn't like you while simultaneously living a life you are proud of, those people who don't like you don't seem to concern you as much. This way of living gives you the freedom to be yourself. What a great gift.

You might believe that when you stop trying to be liked by others, you stop being liked by others. This, however, is far from true as one has nothing to do with the other. In fact, when you give up the need to be liked, you typically end up with better friends because you stop worrying about the people who don't appreciate you and enjoy more of your time with the ones who do. You will probably reduce the overall number of friends you thought you had, but you will improve your relationships with the ones who truly care about you. And they are really the ones worth appreciating.

Those who refuse to be your friends are missing out on knowing someone great. You have a lot to share, and the people who cherish you are going to get to experience that. And yes, that even means that when you appreciate yourself, you get to experience everything great that you are capable of being.

There are several books that address how to make other people like you, but you picked up this book for a different reason. This book is not about getting others to like you but getting you to like who you are.

This world is not fair. You will not get everything you want or always be treated the same as others, but good always comes out of bad. There is a light at the end of the tunnel, but if you sacrifice your principles and morality based on momentary circumstances, you won't see that light because that light shines from within you. It is your perseverance that will push you through all the difficult times, but it is your perspective that determines whether you feel good or bad when all is said and done.

When you lead a good life,
you are always in good company: your own.

Chapter 9

The Significance of Doubt

The journey of overcoming depression, like any undertaking, can at times breed self-doubt. Goals will seem overwhelming and when you don't witness an acceptable amount of progress, you will begin doubting your ability to succeed.

Self-doubt is something that many encounter when striving for a goal or even considering the possibility of achieving some success. As you encounter doubt throughout your life, your motivation skills will be challenged. In order to stay motivated through these times, you will need to continue your physical and mental techniques for keeping your energy high; but you will also need to examine your doubt.

Self-doubt is the feeling of not believing in oneself, and it can affect a number of different aspects of your life. You might doubt your intelligence, attractiveness, talent, experience, or possibly your ability to make a difference. You look at a goal and you look at yourself, and you fear that you don't have it in you to succeed. This leads to the view that it's not even worth trying anymore, often causing you to walk away from what you want most. That's doubt, and it leads to an effortless life of low self-esteem, one of the many characteristics of depression.

Meaning

In a life in which our effort is significant, it's essential to understand why we sometimes doubt its significance. The reason is something called "Delusions of Grandeur." This is the false overestimation of importance. Now you may be questioning how self-doubt could be caused by an abundance of self-confidence. Well, it's not. The delusion of grandeur is specific to the goal, not the person. The cause of doubt is due to giving too much meaning to personal desires.

Whatever you invest your time and focus into is important because you believe that it has some bearing on your life, and it probably does. However, its effect on the rest of your life is probably not as substantial as you believe. People overestimate the significance of tests, assignments, projects, and so many other ambitions all the time. It is rare that something will alter the future dramatically, but how meaningful you view the result will directly affect your confidence in your own abilities.

By building a goal up in your head, you give more significance to the goal than to yourself. By believing that something will have life-changing effects on you, you become paranoid that any wrong move will jeopardize that future. But when you recognize that the results of your failures or successes will not seal your fate in life, you substantially reduce your fears, thereby increasing your chances of persevering past the appearance of doubt.

Don't foresee the results of your actions as the determining steps of your future. Understand that your actions are just what you are choosing to do now. You can't do them for what they will mean to your life, someone else, or even the world. That's too much pressure on anyone.

Think about if you've ever wanted to speak to someone you found attractive but didn't because you doubted the person would be interested in you. Your doubt most likely arose from the belief that the person could play some meaningful role in your life. Believing that one day that person might be a boyfriend/girlfriend or even a spouse suggests that the one action of speaking to that person could play a significant role in your future. And in the fear of messing up what could be, you walked away when the truth is that all you would have been doing is talking to another person; that's it.

Because good advice can often be misunderstood, it's necessary that I clarify what I mean by reducing meaning in your personal desires. I am not suggesting that you eliminate meaning from your life. If you looked at something as meaningless, there wouldn't be any incentive to pursue your goal. Convincing yourself that there was no significance to success would cause you to become stagnant and unmotivated.

Meaning is not the problem but the whole reason to do anything. The problem is simply that people often give things so much meaning that they place their objectives above their capacity. The result of an action can't be everything. The point of reducing the excessive significance of an action's aftermath is to stop yourself from doubting, not to stop yourself from trying.

You give up on yourself because you can't recognize your exact value. Too often we put our desires on a pedestal and ourselves below them. The significance you give to results and the doubt you give to your ability to achieve those results will stop you from doing anything, even being happy.

Since your focus intensifies things, focusing on the result also means focusing on something that doesn't even exist yet. So you end up intensifying the absence of something in your life. That intensification of not yet having what you want makes you question the challenges you face in making it come to be.

Your job is to constantly remind yourself that you are capable of accomplishing what you set out to do. Tell yourself out loud, "I can do this" or "I will do this." Don't do it for what it might create. What matters is that you give your all so that succeed or fail, you gain pride in yourself that you overcame difficulty and doubt to pursue your ambitions.

You have to believe in yourself to accomplish things, but do them because they are what you want to do, not because you believe they will mark the quintessential turning point in your life. Making situations out to be overly substantial puts undue pressure on yourself, causing you to fear, doubt, and give up on what you want.

The fact is that the world will continue to turn whether you succeed or fail. Good will result over time no matter what happens, but your goals have to be attainable. Goals become too large when they have too much meaning. No one thing determines the course of your entire life. In fact, most of your goals only address the next step of your life. So treat them that way.

Your life has meaning. The things you do have meaning. But all that exists is now. Giving an abundance of meaning to something that does not yet exist is looking blindly into the future while disregarding the significance of what you are doing now.

Don't Believe in the Situation; Believe in Yourself

Sometimes doubt comes at the initial consideration of effort, such as when you consider taking on a new challenge. However, other times, it comes later on after some success has been reached and you question your ability to finish the task. In these cases, goals typically become more involved as you get more involved. In other words, the closer you get to achieving your objective, the more likely you are to raise the bar from what you initially wanted to accomplish to something grander. Maybe you change your deadline, redefine your measure of success, or expand the scope of your desire; you lose sight of the original intention as you consider what the activity could mean for your future.

Suppose, for example, that you set out to run a marathon. As you trained and got faster, you might consider the possibility of winning the marathon. This consideration could lead to thoughts of what wining the race would mean for you as an athlete. And as the significance of winning the race built up in your head, you lost the initial desire to just run a marathon and replaced it with the desire to win the marathon. This transformation of desire from possible to delusional is a catalyst for doubt. It is entirely possible that you could win the marathon. However, if you train with the belief that you must win, not only is there only one possible outcome that will make you happy; but you will also doubt your own abilities anytime you encounter struggle. Running a marathon is difficult enough, as are many tasks that we take on in our own lives. And as the significance of a goal grows, so does your doubt.

Technique: Reconnecting with Yourself

If your intentions continuously become more elaborate before you succeed at your original intention, you will never succeed. Success will always be just out of reach. And when you focus on what you have not yet achieved, you will likely see yourself as the reason for not meeting your goals. You discredit yourself, possibly losing interest in your goals and often giving up on everything you have already accomplished.

While your past is never as important as what you are doing in this moment, it's essential that you give yourself credit for what you have done rather than resentment for what you haven't done. You do this by thinking back to what you first wanted to achieve and why you wanted to achieve it.

Instead of developing new intentions and focusing on how far away a goal might be, by reconnecting with your original intention, you realize how far you've come. In doing that, you redistribute meaning from your ambitions to yourself. This gives you pride in yourself and confidence in your abilities. It puts the significance of a goal where it rightfully belongs: on you (because only by believing in yourself can you pursue your goals to completion).

Reconnecting with your original intention doesn't mean you can't develop the depth of your goals; it just means that you must learn to crawl before you can walk. Your knowledge and abilities are each built upon your effort and experiences. And if you skip the effort part of life, you won't have the knowledge and abilities to get you to the next step.

When you get wrapped up in goals, you can get lost. However, thinking back to your original intention can actually give you the important insight you need in order to know how to achieve the goals in front of you. By getting in touch with why you started pursuing something in the first place, you remember what initially mattered to you. And if you now focus on what once drove your interest in something, the path of what to do can often become clear.

———

This technique is not called "Reconnecting with Your Original Intention"; it is called "Reconnecting with Yourself" because it helps you to befriend the person you are. When we doubt ourselves, we are not friendly to ourselves. We look down on our abilities. We criticize ourselves, are disappointed with our performance, and many times give up on an objective because of a lack of faith in our capabilities. But think about how you really motivate yourself in life. The importance of effort cannot be overstated because so many of us our not truly working hard in order to do our best; we are working hard to get to the end of projects. We are often rushing through challenges and forcing ourselves to be better than we have been in the past simply to get to a result. Working hard is important, but if your effort is only sustained by what you are working toward, your doubt in yourself may just be your way of rebelling against yourself.

It's important to give yourself credit for more than just your accomplishments; it's essential that you also pat yourself on the back for the way you live your life. When you doubt, you've forgotten why you started pursuing your objectives. You've lost your way and your confidence because of your need to succeed. You've started focusing on the wrong reasons to accomplish your aspirations: the reward. Forget about all those results that don't really matter. Give it your best shot because that's all that you can ask of yourself. And really, that's all that matters.

The idea that you have to achieve something monumental can be overwhelming. Whether or not you have made some huge contribution to the world or made something grand of yourself doesn't mean that what you are doing isn't important. I mean you are reading a book to help improve your life. That's a pretty big deal, and you should give yourself credit for the effort you're making. Be proud of yourself. Not everyone does this. You're on the road to a better life because it's important to you and it, therefore, has meaning. If you fail to see the meaning in what you do but emphasize the meaning in what you have not yet succeeded at, you'll always be unsatisfied and doubt yourself.

Stop believing that you have to be perfect. It's not all it's cracked up to be. In fact, there's only one direction to go from perfection: down. You're failures and successes do not mean anything definitive about you. Put your meaning squarely on your effort because that is what you are doing. That is what has value. You are what you do, be it simple or grand. And truthfully, if you can't be happy leading a simple life, you'll never be happy leading a grand life; and the reverse is also true.

When you are lost on how to proceed and ready to give up because you feel the journey is unattainable, try a different approach to your objective. Assuming you will not be disrespectful or hurting someone, pick a method, any method to reach your goal. Usually down the line, you will figure out an effective way for you to succeed. You may discover that your new path works, or you may discover that it's necessary to start all over; but at least you will have discovered how to achieve your aim.

Your own personal path has probably not been as easy or as flawless as you would have liked it to be. But when you find consistent happiness in your life, will you really care how long or difficult the process was to reach that point? All that will matter is that you made the effort. It is your unwavering belief in your ability to pursue your goals with skill and commitment that makes accomplishing your goals possible.

Instant Gratification

In the way the world works today, you can find out almost anything with the touch of a button; you can rewind a television show if the commercials weren't long enough for your bathroom break, and you can email someone your business report through your phone. Technology has offered many advances that simplify life, but it has also given rise to the expectancy that things can happen as soon as you decide you want them to happen. It has become exceedingly easy to accomplish so many tasks that any feelings of struggle or needing more time can feel like failure.

With the speed of information, we are also often exposed to the success of others. Every "overnight success" took years of work, but many of us do not understand that. We are only exposed to one aspect of their lives: their success. On the other hand, we are exposed to every aspect of our own lives. So we see the challenges, the time, and the effort we have made. This false impression of reality can leave you questioning why others are succeeding with ease while you are not. Struggle can then be misinterpreted as meaning something is wrong with you personally, causing you to doubt and give up on yourself.

Too many people quit what they do because they don't see results instantly. People tend to switch jobs often. Divorce is common. There is little loyalty anymore, including the loyalty people have to themselves. But loyalty isn't just consideration; it's a commitment, and it is important because without that commitment, there isn't enough time to enjoy the fruits of your labor. Few things seem to be worth the effort because few people realize how much effort it really takes to achieve goals.

To make changes in your life, be it to overcome depression or fulfill any other ambition, will take time, effort, and patience. It is your effort coupled with taking the time needed to achieve your ambitions that allows them to materialize, but it is your patience that allows you to continue putting forth effort over that time period. If you go through life believing the false notion that work should be easy and yield speedy results, you will misinterpret every sign of struggle as a sign of failure and consequently doubt yourself.

Being in a rush to get to the end of a project will not allow you to be satisfied because there never really is an end. Every result leads to something else. I know it feels better to rush through the rough spots to get to where you want to be, but the journey from desire to result is where you learn. It is the effort that makes you who you are, and creating your life is a process that takes time—one small, realistic step at a time.

Worrying

Because results are not instantaneous, the time you spend waiting to finish projects, deal with issues, and get answers can sometimes eat away at you. And while doubt comes from magnifying the impact of success, worry comes from magnifying the impact of failure.

So often we do not just focus on the opportunities that lie before us; we also focus on the possibilities of what could happen if we fail in our aspirations. Worry involves the belief that failure will make your life worse off. You might believe that failure would leave you humiliated, let down someone else, or give up opportunities. This fear of what failure would mean for you causes you to place your skepticism squarely on your own effort to overcome any hardships that failing might trigger. So you intensify the value of failure while reducing the value of your own effort.

Whether you doubt that you will succeed or worry that you will fail, both emphasize a future that has not yet happened. And just as the past can divert your focus and prevent you from moving on, the future can do the same.

When you worry, you emotionally deal with a negative situation before it even turns negative. However, there is no preparation in worry; there is only turmoil. Even if a situation does turn out badly, worrying ahead of time only means that you suffer the emotional distress twice: once based on the thought and a second time based on reality. You stress yourself out, and it doesn't have any effect on the results you worry about. It only makes you feel uncomfortable every moment that you fear how you will live your life once something goes downhill.

Life's too short to waste your energy. Exploring your experiences so that you can understand, address, and predict the likelihood of an outcome gives you insight into life. But magnifying the significance of what you don't yet know to be true only takes you away from this moment. It makes it impossible to address your concerns because your mind is elsewhere. It's focusing on everything that could go wrong when nothing you are worried about has yet to go wrong.

When you feel like there is nothing you can do to help solve a concern, stop looking outward to solve the problem that is affecting your emotions; instead, look inward and focus on solving how you feel. Explore your feelings, asking questions and providing yourself answers so that you can understand your worry. Understanding often leads to acceptance, which brings your emotions down to a tolerable level where worry does not exist. And then you will have solved the problem most affecting you: how you feel.

Blame

Your own doubt about whether you can succeed is not always exclusive to your view of yourself. While self-doubt is the belief that you are incapable of accomplishing a goal, many people commonly accuse something outside themselves for causing their weaknesses. Some people blame the goal for being unnecessarily difficult; some blame others for causing them to have to solve a dilemma, and some blame those who don't believe in their abilities. Occasionally some people will even go so far as to blame the encouragement of others. How could this be?

Assume that you are working hard for a goal, and someone who cares about you believes in your ability to succeed. But then you put so much significance into what you want to accomplish that you end up doubting your own ability and quit putting forth effort. Since your loved one believed in you and you came to doubt yourself and give up, you might feel as though your loved one was wrong for believing in you. By being wrong about something that has left you where you don't want to be, that encouraging person can seem like the obvious one to blame for your failure. So you take the burden of failure off of yourself by blaming someone who believed in you in order to avoid the depression of having given up. You replace your sadness with anger. This is one of the big reasons why children often argue with loving parents.

It doesn't matter who outside yourself believes or doesn't believe in your abilities. Whatever or whomever you look to blame in times of doubt, you are the one who decides what you can and can't do. It is you who has to look past all the distractions in your life and decide for yourself at this place and time what to set out to do with your life—and then do it or don't.

What does it mean if you believe in yourself, don't succumb to doubt, follow through, and still fail? It means that there are other factors at work in this world besides you. Every relationship, including the relationship between you and your objectives, is dependent on two ingredients: the right people and the right circumstances. Only when these two aspects of a relationship continue to sync up will a relationship flourish.

In this world, certain chemicals are combined to create life while others create explosions. Some people find themselves in love but on different paths. Some climates are too cold for one species while too hot for another. Everyone is different and situations are constantly changing, making what might be right for you at one time not right for you at another time. However, you only discover which relationships work and which don't when you put forth effort.

Sometimes you will look at your life and see a lot of work in your path. Under the surface, you may feel frustrated by failure or scared by pressure to be a certain way or accomplish a certain goal. Life, however, takes time; and what keeps you going is not being demanding of yourself but knowing why you are doing something.

We often make things out to be bigger than they are. We believe that success or failure will signify our own importance in this world, affect how others view us, and be a catalyst for positive change or a sign that disappointment is imminent. But truthfully, it doesn't mean any of these. Your life is constantly changing and is represented at each moment by what you chose to do with it. So make your life based on doing things that you believe in, not based on avoiding things you doubt.

When you overanalyze situations,
you doubt your own ability to handle them.

Chapter 10

The Fate of Hope

Let me tell you what I want. I want to be awake in this world, receptive to all that is around me, interacting with others I encounter. I want to smell the roses around me rather than dream of different roses far away. I want to appreciate all that I have rather than wish for everything I don't have. I want to look around and smile rather than lower my gaze and cry. I want to listen to what people are saying rather than think about what I'll say once they're done speaking. I want to accept what's happening rather than fear what might come. I want to take a deep breath and breathe this air in front of me rather than hold my breath until what I want to happen comes true. I want to be at peace rather than waiting for a verdict.

This is what I want. Maybe it's what you want too. What I do know is that the only way to kick depression is by making the most of what exists in this moment right now because it's the only thing that is real. Your doubt stems from you giving more meaning to your goals than to your abilities; you essentially focus on something that doesn't exist. In this same way, many of the beliefs you may have about hope can similarly lead you to place significance on a future that may never come to be.

Throughout your life, you have probably heard ideals about hope. Many great leaders have spoken about the power of hope, but hope can be a dangerous thing if it's all you have. If you place your happiness on a hope, you are gambling with your emotions. If that hope doesn't come true, it can feel like losing everything even though you never lost anything.

Let's examine hope. When you say that you hope something ends up a certain way, what you mean is that you will be happy *if* a situation results in the way you desire. So with hope, you focus on the result of the future, discrediting the importance of what you have in your life now. It is not hope, however, that causes you to lose sight of the good things that exist in your life. Rather, losing sight of those good things is what causes you to hope.

When you fail to see the good you have in your life, holding on to hope provides the belief that what you want is not far off. Hope makes you feel as though your emotional attachment to what you want is keeping it alive as a possibility. But hope creates instability in your life. From the moment you begin hoping for an outcome, you put your life in limbo, awaiting a result. Until that result comes, you will worry, imagine, doubt, and experience a plethora of emotions based on a possibility, not a reality. You idly hold back your life, hoping things will turn in your favor. And as you continuously focus on your hopes, giving them more and more intensity, you distract yourself from the present and risk the feeling of devastation if what you want doesn't happen.

Hope has one purpose: to die. In the end, a hope must become a reality or be let go of as a lost cause. The indefinite existence of a hope means that you are waiting, likely waiting impatiently, for your happiness to come around when that future you desire brings it around. Hope, which many believe is keeping them going, may actually be holding them back. It may be causing them to avoid making the most of today by fantasizing about a future they believe is better than now.

Hope is a wish, and wishing for things to be different doesn't make them so. You can't get everything you want in life, but if you look around at what you have and consider what is important to you, you can find so much to appreciate and realize there are things in your life that are more worthy of your attention than your hopes.

The Missing Link Is Effort

Don't get me wrong; there is something beautiful about hope, but it's empty. It's missing something. It's missing your effort to pursue it to a reality or to accept things as they are. When you hope, you're not doing anything with your life other than anxiously waiting for something to occur that will put your anxiety to rest.

You must not be a bystander in the act of hoping but a participant in extinguishing that hope. Hope can provide you valuable insight into knowing what you want. The trick is that once you recognize what you want, rather than putting your focus on what doesn't exist (your hope), put your focus on what does exist (yourself).

Using the "Questions" technique from Chapter 6, recognize why you want what you want. As you learn about yourself, you may find that there are other ways to bring into your life the happiness that you are seeking with a particular hope. You may even find that what you hope for really doesn't matter as much as you thought. It may turn out that what you hope for is really just a means to an end.

Imagine for a moment that through self-exploration regarding your feelings about one of your hopes, you discovered that what you hope for isn't actually the best way to bring into your life what really matters to you. For example, maybe you realized that your hope to be in an intimate relationship with someone specific is really just based on a desire to be loved even though that person isn't actually a good fit for you. Now what if you hadn't done that self-exploration and that hope came true? Because it doesn't hold as much importance as you attributed to it, that hope becoming a reality might not even make you happy. I'm willing to guess that there are many things in life that you have hoped for, but when they came around, you still weren't happy and consequently saw yourself as a victim of depression, thinking that you'd never be happy. The truth is you may just be hoping for things that don't represent what matters to you deep down.

You may, however, discover through self-examination that what you hope for truly does matter to you. If it does, go for it.

What gives hope value is effort and that comes directly from you. If you use your hope to fuel your effort toward pursuing what you want, what you now have in your sight is a goal. By choosing what to do and following through, your hope is no longer your only asset. Remember how I said in chapter 2 that a drug can be used as a tool or as an escape? Hope is very similar. If you use it to fuel your effort, it has a purpose. However, if you just sit around hoping, it only serves as a means of escaping the reality of today.

Some people may question how to know whether there is anything they can do about a situation or if they are just holding on to false hope. Well, hope is only false when it isn't backing your effort because your effort is what makes success possible. However, there are some things in life that just won't happen no matter how much effort you put forth. Paying attention to patterns and being open with communication will give you insight into what, if anything, can actually be done to make your hope a reality.

Many people tend to look at what they hope for and think that they would be willing to put forth effort if there was a chance for success, but because they are not certain about the future, they debate what to do. Truthfully, whether or not you succeed in the end is beside the point. You will never know for sure if you can accomplish what you want until you accomplish it. But rather than focusing on your odds of success, just consider whether what you want is worth your effort. Once you answer that question, you'll have your answer of whether to pursue a hope one step further than this moment.

You are the one who has to be happy with what you do with your life, not just what you get for what you do. I know how strong hope can feel. I know how much it can hurt to give up hope, but if you don't believe you can do anything to make your hope a reality or you just no longer feel that what you are getting out of a situation is worth your effort, it's time to let go of that desire because it is inhibiting you from moving on with your life.

It's time to wake up from the dreams that you call hopes.

It's time to stop waiting for something to make you happy. It's time to look around at what really exists, see what the world is offering, and do something great with what you have in order to give yourself what you truly value. The time to wake up is now because now is what exists. And there is no hope in now. There is only you and your surroundings. That is what is real, and that is what you must accept.

If you don't take action to pursue what you hope for or to move on from it, you'll remain in the waiting room of life with no promise that happiness will ever call your name. This is not something to be sad about because what it really means is that you don't have to wait for happiness. You can have it as soon as you realize that right now might just provide you some great opportunities to make you happy if you take advantage of them.

Expectations

Hope looks beyond this moment. It looks to the future, a future that may or may not come to be. Many times, however, we don't just hope for a particular future; we count on it. This may occur because someone said he/she would do something or even because patterns have shown the probability of things ending up a certain way. These expectations that many of us have about the future can cause the same pain as unfulfilled hope because life doesn't always turn out the way you plan.

A phrase that can often save you from the disappointment of unmet expectations is: "Do not count your chickens before they are hatched."[1] This quote is a reminder that even when a situation seems sure to turn out a particular way, anything can happen. There is no precise way to always be certain about something until you see what transpires.

Setting expectations is jumping ahead of the next step. When you expect a particular future, you plan your life around that future. It becomes the basis for how you act now and how you plan to act once the expectation takes place. However, if the expectation doesn't become a reality, you then have to reevaluate how to live your life. This often leads to a feeling of frustration as you have already accepted an experience before it has happened.

Expectations are most hazardous to your well-being when they involve people because unmet expectations can lead to a loss of confidence in those people. This is even true when it comes to your relationship with yourself. Think about when you don't live up to your own expectations. You lose confidence in yourself. And I'll tell you, if you have expectations about how long it should take you to overcome depression, you might lose confidence in your own ability to overcome the challenges you face at each step. What's that lack of confidence called again? That's right; it's called doubt.

Life happens in steps. That's how you flow with life. If you reject the steps between now and the future, you will disregard all the effort and circumstances between now and then. Remember, a relationship takes the right people and the right circumstances, which means that your future happening the way you expect is not just dependent on your effort and the effort of others but the circumstances you both encounter. Too often though, we mistake the impact of those circumstances for a lack of personal effort, which can play negatively on our relationships and our self-esteem.

Having plans is good, but you must be flexible. If you close yourself off from the possibility of change, you will be unprepared for life whenever your anticipations are not met. Let people live their lives just as they allow you to live yours. You must be open to the possibility that what you thought would happen can change without letting it ruin your day or shatter your world. So have a backup plan called confidence in yourself.

Expectation Spectrum

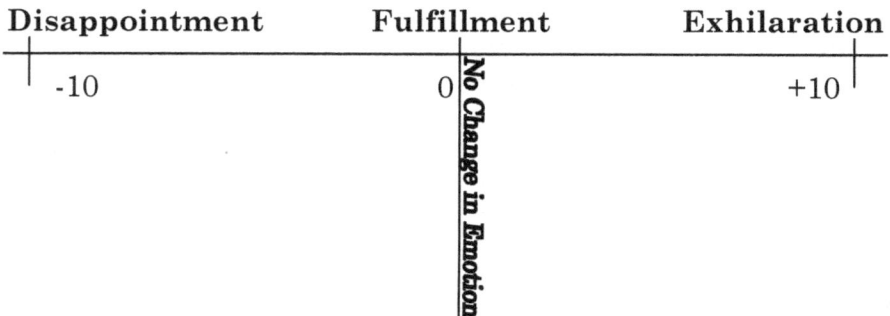

Disappointment	Fulfillment	Exhilaration
-10	0	+10

No Change in Emotion

Take a look at the Expectation Spectrum diagram. When you set up an expectation, you perceive your life with a specific future. If the future goes exactly as you anticipate, your expectation would be fulfilled and you wouldn't be affected dramatically. You knew it would happen that way and, therefore, have no change in emotion.

If, however, you set an expectation for the future and it is not fulfilled, your emotions will fall into the negative numbers and you will encounter a feeling of disappointment. In fact, the more significance you place on your expectation, the more disappointment you will feel if it goes unfulfilled.

On the other end of the spectrum are positive numbers, which you move into when you get something more than you anticipate. Since you don't expect anything extra, you secure a feeling of exhilaration. Do you see the problem here? The only way you can get that feeling of exhilaration is from getting benefits, on top of fulfillment, that you don't expect. In reality, however, when you expect something, you almost always get either fulfillment or fall short of that. This means that the Expectation Spectrum rarely has a scale of +10 to -10; it almost always has a scale of 0 to -10.

Many people on the road to depression have high expectations. And over time, repeated experiences of getting less than they expected cause them to lose faith in this world. They then put forth less effort toward what they want while holding low expectations, essentially waiting for bad things to happen.

When you are depressed, you expect that people won't keep their word, things will go wrong, and the worst will happen. Based upon looking at the Expectation Spectrum, you might assume that this way of looking at life would create exhilaration often since the bar for fulfillment would be set so low. The problem with this way of thinking is that every moment you spend waiting for a result is filled with despair. You never put forth effort because you don't believe that good things are possible, and without effort, your life is completely out of your control.

Understanding these problems with having high or low expectations, you might set out to avoid having any expectations at all. Many people actually believe in living a life without expectations. However, bouncing to the extreme of not having expectations can actually lead to depression just as easily as having high or low expectations. This is because expectations suggest some degree of personal importance in something taking place. If you didn't expect the possibility of something occurring, you wouldn't try. For example, if someone said he/she would meet you at a certain place and time but you didn't expect that person to show up, you wouldn't be there to meet him/her. Therefore, not having any expectations would stop you from doing anything because everything would be pointless. So what is one to do?

Many people have high expectations, low expectations, or no expectations because they don't see any other option, leaving them repeatedly disappointed. However, there is a fourth option: "Moderate Expectations." Somewhere between having high and low expectations is a balance in which you don't anticipate the best or the worst. You have faith but are open to the possibility that things might not work out.

But where is the dividing line that separates high and low expectations? The answer to this involves not focusing on which expectations are too high or too low but *understanding the consequences* of high and low expectations. When you set your expectations too high, you aren't open to change. When you set your expectations too low, you aren't open to trusting others. So by learning to be open to change *and* how to trust people, you avoid the extremes of expectations and instead create moderate expectations in your life. Let's first examine how to prepare for unexpected changes to your expectations, essentially not expecting perfection.

Prepare for the Possibilities

The way to avoid setting expectations too high is to be open to a change in circumstances, but how can you be open to change when expectation conveys a certainty? The way to set plans while remaining prepared for change is through two steps. The first step is, once again, to limit how much meaning you give to the fulfillment of your expectation. This is important because giving too much meaning to an expectation puts your focus on the result, which is out of your hands. The second step is to consider the possibilities of what else might happen besides what you expect. This way, you are prepared to move on rather than getting upset if what you expect does not occur.

An example of preparing for the possibilities would be if I bought a computer. I would expect that it would work (otherwise I wouldn't buy it), but if I were to consider the possibility that it might fail at some point, I could adequately prepare myself now for that. One example would be to back up my data regularly.

In life, when you believe something is one way, don't remain tied to it. Appreciate it, but know that anything can change; and if it does change, it's not the end of the world. When you prepare for change, the impact of that change is substantially lessened. The fact is that all the problems you have in your life are only considered problems because you weren't prepared for them, and they only remain problems until you handle them. It is your openness and preparation for potential change that allows you to avoid the frustration of things not working out the way you hoped or expected.

Trust
When you prepare for change, your expectations don't hold as much significance; and you consequently don't set your expectations too high. But to avoid setting your expectations too low, you must have some faith in their ability to come true. This is where trust comes into play.

Trust is an aspect of security (a basic human need), but being open to change seems to contradict the ability to believe someone's word.[2] The problem for many is that they do not distinguish between trusting and expecting. However, the fine line between trust and expectation is, not surprisingly, effort.

Trust of others is based on their intentions. When you don't trust people, you believe they have ill intentions. When you do trust them, you believe that their intentions are in line with their commitments. Because it is the intention that determines trustworthiness, when someone puts forth effort to honor his/her commitment, that person proves he/she is trustworthy regardless of whether the end result is what was intended. What matters is the respect someone has for you, and that is displayed by effort, not outcome.

Consider a situation in which someone promised to pick you up but cancelled at the last minute because of a family emergency. Your expectation would have been that the person would pick you up while your trust would have been that the person had consideration for you. This hypothetical situation wouldn't be a breach of trust because the intention of the person did not change. Things happen and get in the way of people's commitments, but the effort, rather than the end result, is what matters. Don't expect results to always represent your trust.

People typically say that trust is earned, meaning that trust is only gained when someone consistently proves to be reliable. This statement is only perceived to be true because if someone always comes through on promises, it suggests that the person is putting forth effort into his/her commitments. However, reliability of result cannot be the determining factor in trust because people's intentions may not always be displayed in the same manner. You may be treated different ways by the same people throughout your life, but as long as those actions always come from the same place of respect, trust must remain. It is when the intentions behind the actions change that there is cause to reevaluate the relationship.

When you focus on the effort, you have trust. When you focus on the end result, you have expectation. By relying on results to prove trustworthiness, you create expectations of people that they then have to live up to. This puts your relationships in a vulnerable position because if someone has been consistently reliable, failure to continue this trend will cause you to stop trusting the person. It is a person's intentions that truly display whether he/she is trustworthy. Have you ever heard the expression "It's the thought that counts"? It's true.

Since intentions are internal, it can be difficult to know the reasoning behind people's actions. This is why so many people rely on results to determine whether they can trust others. While patterns of past results can give an indication of the future, so can patterns of past intentions. Therefore, the best way to figure out the reasoning behind another's actions is simply to ask and listen closely. It's not essential that the person's intentions were to solely make you happy but that your feelings were at least considered in a situation in which you were involved.

What you have to realize when you check in with others' intentions is that just because you believe you're involved in a situation doesn't always means that others think you're involved. And why would people consider someone's feelings whom they didn't think was involved in a situation? They wouldn't, and they don't. Just because you have a vested interest in something doesn't always mean you are involved. In any situation, it is only when someone knows a person is involved *and* completely disregards that person's feelings in which trust is truly broken.

It is true that sometimes a person will lie in order to avoid confrontation, hurting another's feelings, or admitting guilt; but you cannot assume anything beyond what you know to be true. You either believe the person or you don't. However, if you don't believe what someone tells you, the problem is not how that person treated you; it is how you view that person. The issue of trust being broken is beside the point. The fact is that if you don't believe what you are told, you already don't trust that person; and the relationship is doomed.

A common practice is that people will not trust others but look for ways to trust them. For example, I've known of people who suspected their lovers were cheating on them; and in an effort to confirm their suspicions, they spied on them. They believed that if they discovered that their lovers were being faithful, they could then trust them. However, what they failed to realize was that whether or not their lovers were cheating on them didn't really matter. The real problem was that their lovers' behavior made them so uncomfortable that they didn't trust them.

Trying to trust people based on results alone is not possible. You either trust them or you don't. But without trust, you cannot feel secure in your relationships; and they cannot be sustained. It will be your ability to see the intentions behind actions that provide you the insight into whether you can trust certain people. Beyond that, all that exists are results; and they don't amount to much.

When you trust intentions but are open to change, your expectations no longer hold your happiness hostage. This is how you create moderate expectations in your life. What you hope for or expect to happen in life doesn't always happen. But when you prepare for the possibility of change, you protect your relationship with yourself. When you learn to trust others' intentions, you protect your relationships with others.

Recognizing patterns and being open with communication will help you determine whether you can trust assurances you are given. But your own effort to prepare for the possibilities that can come with change eases the impact of disappointment when those assurances don't materialize into the results you expect.

As with everything in life, it is how you interact with the world around you that affects your experiences. But those interactions do not occur down the road somewhere. They are constantly occurring in how you handle yourself every step of the way until what you hope or expect to happen takes place or doesn't.

We live in one moment and this is it right now. And when you focus on a future that may never come around, you miss out on this moment. You have so much to appreciate and utilize around you, but focusing on your life in the future will almost never pay you back the energy you need to feel good about yourself. It is your hopes and expectations that shift your focus from what exists in your life to what doesn't exist. You give up the opportunity to be happy now for the chance that the future holds a different reason to be happy.

Anything can happen in this world, but what makes a hope possible is effort. What makes a hope acceptable is the willingness to be able to live without that hope becoming a reality. If right now, you can look around and not see anything good in your life, your eyes are closed. You are focusing on something that isn't real. Maybe it's a wish, a regret, or something you didn't get. It doesn't matter. What matters is taking what you have today and making the most of it. And that's truly how you create the better tomorrow you hope for.

Everything except now is just a thought.

Chapter 11

The Only Constant Is Change

Human beings have survived millions of years because they have evolved in relation to their surroundings.[1] Similarly, your own willingness to adapt to the world around you is central to whether your life feels like a struggle or an opportunity. One of the biggest mistakes you can make is becoming complacent, believing that your life will forever remain the way it is at this very moment.

Both self-doubt and hope can lead to feelings of worthlessness and unease because they involve basing your happiness on a future that may never come. They dismiss reality as it exists in this moment. Hope and doubt center around one thing: the future. And the future promises just one thing: change.

Everything in this world changes at some point. Friends change, events change, plans change, and even you change. Because change is inevitable, you are guaranteed that nothing in your life will last forever. Jobs will end, people will die, and the present will become the past. Nothing is a sure thing except change. Evidence suggests probability, but change is the one constant in life.

As discussed earlier, one of the reasons we hold on to patterns is fear of the unknown. When you grow accustomed to a way of life, you find comfort in the way things are even if it's not the best way of living. When you are forced to endure a change to that way of life, even if it could be beneficial, a change to comfort is typically interpreted as discomfort.

Everyone who is alive right now has survived everything that has come into their lives up to this very moment. However, instead of acknowledging their ability to overcome adversity, many see the unknown as something that could possibly destroy what they have. This negative way of thinking leads to anxiety, anger, and even prejudice.

Refusing to change with your surroundings is a substantial contributor to what makes people depressed. It is why so many people who are depressed compare their current circumstances to a more favorable past. They are holding on to what is gone and, therefore, literally holding on to nothing. And how can you be happy when you view what you currently have as worse than nothing?

People talk about "the good old days," but the truth is the good old days weren't so good. There were problems in the past that don't exist now. People only look back and glorify the past when they encounter new inconveniences. They fail to see all the good that has resulted from change since the good old days. The benefit of that change, however, is called progress.

The progress that we have made as a human race is built on the collective intelligence of everyone who has come before us. While the progress of humanity has not come without its share of problems, society is better than it once was in many ways. Similarly, as every situation changes, it brings many great aspects with it. It won't all be perfect. Some parts of a new experience may be more difficult than past ones. But by accepting what comes along, you evolve and are able to survive the experience. And that is our most basic human goal: survival.[2]

Change happens every day, and the more you oppose it, the harder it will be to feel good. You will feel as though life is always shitting on you. It's not shitting on you though; it's changing and your reaction is hostile. You likely haven't taken the time to evaluate your circumstances for benefits. And when you are unappreciative, you are unhappy, condemning the change to your life that replaced what you once had, even if you only had it briefly.

Change, however, does not need to be resisted so fiercely. By accepting that everything changes, you gain many opportunities. The realization that change is imminent means that hard times in your life will always come to an end. It also means that good times will likewise cease, reminding you to appreciate what you have in the moment as it is fleeting.

No matter if an experience at any given time feels pleasant or painful, it is real in that moment. It is the acceptance of that reality that allows you to make the most of life. It is the acceptance that there is something to gain from that experience that makes it truly valuable. But it is also the acceptance that situations will change, others will change, and you will change that prepares you for these changes.

When you oppose what you encounter in this world, you become a victim, arguing back at a world that you feel is causing you problems. This fight against what has already happened can literally feel overwhelming as you focus on how something or someone held you back from what is important to you. Ironically, what is holding you back is actually your opposition of it. The passionate belief that the way things used to be held significance and circumstances being different means a significant problem for you is what makes life feel uneasy. It is only when you embrace something that it feels just right.

There are some things in life that you simply cannot change. What you can change, however, is how you integrate with this world. And as you do this, you are no longer the subject of change; you are the instigator of change.

Let Go with the Flow

Imagine you held your finger so tight that you cut off the circulation. You would be stopping the natural flow of blood through your finger. The longer you kept the blood from moving on, the worse off your finger would become, turning cold and losing feeling. Similarly in life, you may often be causing yourself harm by trying to stop situations from changing.

You may feel as though if you refuse to move on from the past, your surroundings will return to the way they were. But holding on to what once existed only makes the pain of change linger. You may argue, criticize, or complain because you feel like you are being treated unfairly. But as you oppose changes to what you had, you focus exclusively on what's wrong with your life.

Just like hoping for a future that doesn't exist, resisting change is hoping for a return of the past, which too no longer exists. When you refuse to accept change, you let the past control you. When you accept change, you control what you do with the present.

Let's examine this a bit more so that you understand exactly how much control you gain from accepting life as it is. Let's say that you were fired from your job. If you were to oppose this and fight it, you would feel the disappointment of change being forced upon you. You might complain or cry, feeling as though you were at the whim of life's changes. Your life would become stagnant as you focused on your detriment.

Now say that as soon as you were fired, you chose to accept this reality, possibly thinking how you might be better off without the job. Rather than demanding or pleading for the lost cause of regaining your job or getting angry at your former employer, you recognize that you can't do anything about your job loss and instead focus your energy on finding a new job or using your newfound free time to work on a project. By accepting the reality of your predicament, you instantly gain the ability to move on from the situation. You understand that your job never controlled you and that you can survive just fine without it. You gain confidence in your ability to succeed in new circumstances.

You may suspect that allowing situations to change without having some say in how they change is a surefire way for people to take advantage of you. You might believe that this way of living will make you a passive observer rather than a proactive individual, but it is quite the contrary. I am not encouraging you to sit on the sidelines as life goes by but simply not block the flow of life. Your role in any change is what you do with your life in the changed circumstances.

Consider how often it is that the things that upset you are due to you resisting change. The truth is that most of the changes you encounter aren't really that big of a deal. The faster you just accept what you encounter, the faster you can figure out what you can do with yourself in this changed world and the faster you can move past any feelings of negativity to actually feeling good about your life. Imagine something bad happening and being able to let it go without letting it bother you. How good would that feel?

Technique: Supporting Reality

When something changes that affects the way you feel, it means that you change, at least temporarily. Your mood, your views, and your confidence are altered. You are given a new reality in which you must now respond. But what truly makes accepting change so difficult is not knowing what to do with yourself in the new circumstances.

When you encounter change that you don't like, the fastest way to accept it is to give your support toward part of the change. Like the political adage "If you can't beat them, join them," it is your support that surrenders your opposition because you can't logically be against something you support.

Now let's be real. In many ways, it seems ridiculous to support something you are against. This is why I said to support "part" of the change. Say, for instance, that your child has developed a drug problem. Obviously, you wouldn't want to support your child's addiction; but there is a very important part of the situation that needs your support: your child. By showing your support for that person, you play an active role in the change you are against.

In a world of change, you will not like everything you experience. You don't have to like everyone you know or everything you have done. But what allows you to get to acceptance so that you can move on is using your energy in a positive sense to extinguish the pain of a negative change. There is good and bad in everything and when you take the time to understand what is good about anything in life and you give your support to that, you recognize how to handle yourself in the changes you oppose. In fact, sometimes the good in a bad situation is simply knowing that you can handle it.

———

Change Is Happening Now

It is not just important to be able to accept change once it has taken place but also to identify change that is occurring right now. Change does not always happen suddenly; it can occur subtly over time. Think about when you are around someone regularly. You rarely notice that person's physical changes as he/she gets older, but when you see people you haven't seen in years, they often look completely different than you remember. A little change every day adds up to a lot.

Subtle changes can sometimes lead to damaging effects over time if those changes are not noticed early on. Many people end up getting divorced because they failed to recognize changes occurring in their spouses. The truth is people and circumstances are always changing around you, and it's up to you to take notice of those changes.

Particularly when you are looking for patterns in life, subtle changes become more obvious. This identification can help you prepare for more significant change on the horizon. And as discussed in the previous chapter, your preparation allows you to be open to change.

Technique: Checking in on Change

Think about the aspects of your relationships that you believe are permanent. Then take the time to ask the people with whom you have those relationships how they feel about the different parts of your relationships, particularly the parts that you are the most confident about. Get to know their perspectives. You will often create better relationships this way. Other times, you may discover that their perspectives differ from your own and that certain relationships are unlikely to last. In either case, you will gain the insight to prepare yourself for possible changes to your relationships.

Your exploration into your relationships will help in making you aware of where things stand, but what you discover will also not permanently hold true. Because change is a constant, even people's perspectives about their relationships will change over time—including yours. Therefore, it is important to regularly explore your relationships.

———

While change is always taking place, sometimes circumstances were always a particular way, only you weren't aware of it. For example, your childhood hero may have been exposed as a criminal, causing you to lose respect for that person. The truth is that your hero may have been a criminal for a long time, but when you learned about this, it was your own perspective of that person that changed. The fact is that until you learn about something, nothing truly exists as far as you know.

If you don't pay attention to what is taking place in your life and make the effort to learn about what exists, you may continue to act as you always have and become confused and disheartened when your relationships encounter problems. When anything in your life changes, your interactions change even if you were not behind the change.

Sometimes, however, the changes in your interactions that seem to be caused by others may be partly due to you changing. Just as everything around you is constantly changing, you too are going through changes that can impact your relationships. For example, consider that when you first start a job, you work hard because you are learning how to do your work properly. After a few years, you may get the same amount of work done without as much effort because it became second nature to you. So you may feel like your job has gotten easier or boring, but it is actually you that has changed.

Because you are constantly exposed to yourself, you might not always notice subtle changes taking place in yourself. But just as you must learn to accept changes in the world around you, you must also learn to accept your own changes. You will grow older; you will make mistakes, and you will fail. You will also learn, have positive experiences, and succeed. You will become someone new, but that is not a bad thing. You have many good qualities now and you will have many good qualities in the future, new ones you may never have thought you would possess. But if you refuse to accept changes to yourself, all you will create for yourself is the feeling of pressure.

Looks Can Be Deceiving

One of the big reasons we often have a difficult time accepting change is because what has changed in character sometimes still looks the same physically. Just because events, people, logos, or situations look the same as they did in the past does not mean they are the same. You may be in love with someone who has changed even though he/she still looks like the person you fell in love with long ago. And while it is difficult to separate the person's physicality from personality, that person is no longer who he/she once was.

Let's say that you were dating someone who ended the relationship with you. You might want that person who left you to take you back, but that person is not who you dated. That person is who broke up with you. The person may look the same as who you were dating, but he/she is different.

It is hard enough to accept a change when you've grown accustomed to the way things were. It can be even harder to accept that change when physical appearances seem unchanged because what you see and what you experience are no longer in sync. What can ease the difficulty of this type of situation is the understanding that what you are longing for is not simply out of reach; it is out of existence. What you are seeking is gone, and it won't exhibit the same attributes it once did because it isn't the same as it used to be.

Despite the veil of a physical association we've come to know, what we see is not always what exists. When you realize that with change, you often fight for what is already gone, acceptance comes just a little bit easier than if there was a chance that you could get things back to the way they used to be.

Commitment

The obvious debate that ensues from the realization that change is certain is if you can ever plan for the future or make any sort of commitment. *You certainly can.*

A commitment is a guarantee or pledge of one's loyalty. People make commitments because they don't want their lives to change, and this is exactly what a commitment accomplishes. While change is inevitable over time, a commitment allows a situation to exist longer than it would otherwise. However, something else happens when you make a commitment; you create a relationship.

People get married, sign contracts, and make promises because without these commitments, they would hastily move on from one experience to the next, never getting to explore the depths of their relationships. It is the effort they make to keep someone or something in their lives that allows them to gain a deeper understanding of whom or what they are committing to as well as a deeper understanding of themselves in relation to another. Change will certainly occur in all relationships, but it is the understanding and acceptance of someone or something that allows people to develop alongside those changes rather than seeing any change as a threat to the whole relationship.

While the commitments you make might not last forever, avoiding commitment will ensure that you only scratch the surface of your experiences. You won't get to know the depth of anything in this world unless you commit yourself to an objective. It is your dedication that stabilizes you in a moment long enough so that you can explore, identify, and experience the full possibilities of something, including the way it changes. Being open to change is not the same as avoiding stability.

It is your own failure to commit to making the most of your life that has consequently failed to create a healthy relationship between you and this world. And so you are at odds with your surroundings. However, when you commit to a relationship with your surroundings, you begin to learn about how the world works and how you interact with this world. It's exactly how I learned everything you are reading about in this book. And it's exactly what you will continue to learn by making that same commitment to exploring and making the most of everything you encounter. Commitments are not only possible in a world of change; they are essential.

Change is unavoidable. It is always happening, even right now. You are changing; the people around you are changing, and this world is changing. I know it can be scary. It seems to imply that everything you have worked for, everything you have, and everything you know is only temporary and that it could all be different tomorrow.

Change can feel painful because it is a loss. It is the loss of what was familiar. And in a life in which you create patterns to react to your surroundings, a change in those surroundings can feel jarring. But a change outside of yourself requires a change internally so that you can move forward. Without that internal change, your refusal to accept a new reality can cause you to put your life on hold, hoping the world will return to the way it was. But it never goes back to exactly the way it was. This world always moves on, and so must you.

But who's to say that something different is bad? Who's to say that those changes won't be improvements to what currently exists in your life? Who's to say that what you didn't plan for isn't exactly what you need? With each new situation comes opportunity. It just takes some exploration, acceptance, and action to get you to appreciation.

Change exists for you to learn about yourself. Wherever you go and whatever you encounter, this world is not here so much for you to learn about your surroundings but to learn about yourself in those surroundings. Understanding comes from exploration; freedom comes from acceptance, and growth comes from applying both to your life.

Accept the change you encounter and create the change you want.
That's how you make the most of what you have.

Chapter 12

The Path of Extremism

Accepting change in your life means accepting when things don't go your way, but many people refuse to accept what they encounter when it goes against what they want. These are the people I call extremists, and believe me, I used to be one for a long time.

Those unsatisfied with life typically live on the ends of the pleasure spectrum. They believe that things are either good or bad, that they either work or don't work. This leads to dramatic shifts in feelings when change occurs. If you have something good in your life and it changes, it instantly becomes bad using this mentality. What you want means the world, and not getting what you want means the end of the world. This is the mentality of an extremist.

Because there is little middle ground in the way extremists think, they often want to get everything they seek or would rather nothing at all. It is my way or the highway, and there is no room for compromise. However, at the same time, extremists are rarely willing to accept not getting what they want. So they fight for what they want—all of it. The problem is that rarely does anyone get the whole of what he/she wants. So extremists are almost always disappointed. They are critical and constantly looking at what they don't have or didn't get.

When you fight over every issue in life, you increase the intensity of and lengthen the time in which you deal with dilemmas. You end up constantly exhausted because you feel like you have to fight for everything you want. You end up constantly unhappy because no middle ground will suffice. You end up constantly missing out on opportunities that pass by as you focus strictly on getting your way. And when all the fighting for what you want has ended, rarely do you even care anymore about what you wanted in the first place. The truth is that when you fight for everything, you lose everything.

The interesting thing about extremism is that while your demands may seem important, they are really secondary to what you are truly seeking. You see, when you make demands, you create spaces in your life that you reserve specifically for the fulfillment of those demands. But every moment that your demands go unfulfilled, you continue to feel the emptiness of those spaces in your life. So extremists fight less for what they want and more to avoid that feeling of emptiness continuing.

When you let go of your demands, however, you open up those empty spaces in your life to be filled by all kinds of new experiences. And while opening up can be scary, it is the fast route to fulfillment. By no longer reserving the emptiness in your life for something specific, those spaces can be filled with anything else, possibly something better than what you initially demanded or even knew existed.

There is a common ideology that everything should be done in moderation. This concept is not entirely accurate because many actions can be damaging even in moderation. However, this concept should be more accurately understood to mean that you should never avoid learning about something because nothing is entirely good or bad. The point of moderation is to sample life, what looks pleasing and what looks displeasing. The experiences you gain from this will allow you to recognize the way things actually are rather than making baseless assumptions about the world. By trying new things, you begin to accept that even what you don't want might not be so bad.

Without this knowledge, you jump from ideal to ideal, believing that your vision of the right way is the only way. Anything extreme will lead you down a bad path, be it religious, political, or even ethical. It pits you against everything that is not the way you believe it should be. It leaves no room for compromise and, therefore, no chance for peace with others who have different points of view.

As it should come as no surprise, extremism puts a strain on relationships. Extremists will wish the best for their friends and the worst for their enemies. When people screw up, extremists see it as monumental rather than simple mistakes or errors in judgment. They demand perfection, and since no one will ever amount to that, over time, extremists reject everyone in their lives for one reason or another.

Through exploration, you learn about this world; but by believing that something different from what you want is entirely bad, it is probable that you are missing out on opportunities every day that would benefit your life. The destiny of extremism is depression. Do you have an extremist mentality?

Technique: Are You an Extremist?

One way of determining whether you have an extremist mentality is asking yourself if you have considered committing suicide anytime recently. Suicide is the ultimate extreme consideration. There's nothing after it. It's the end. If suicide seemed like an option recently, you probably continue to handle several aspects of your life with a degree of extremism.

Another way of determining whether you are living as an extremist is to take note of the language you use when characterizing your circumstances. Do you use words like "always," "never," "everything," and "nothing" to describe your life? Examples include: "This *always* happens to me," "This *$#%! machine *never* works," "You forget *everything*," or "*Nothing ever* goes right."

These types of extreme statements are evidence of an extremist mentality and are not just inaccurate but serve to make you feel that your frustration is justified and that there is no way to solve your problems. When you talk about your life in this way, you also alienate people who might otherwise be willing to work with you on solutions. Addressing your life in extremist language reinforces the false sense of reality that life is always a particular way when the truth is that it's not always like this, but it is now. There is only one constant: change. Everything else is in flux, requiring sacrifice and providing opportunities.

———

In order to overcome extremism, you must let go of the need for life to follow some particular path. You must accept that you might not get what you want or planned for and be okay with that. So begin the process of acceptance by accepting the possibility that what you want out of any specific situation isn't going to happen. When you first entertain this thought, you may feel fear, sadness, or even sick to your stomach. But try not to concentrate on how not getting what you want feels. It doesn't take a genius to know that not getting what you want doesn't feel good. Instead, consider what you would do with yourself if what you want in life doesn't happen. Think of some of the big things.

Do you have any major goals in your life? Do you have relationships that mean the world to you? Don't give up on them, but think about what you might do if your future doesn't end up the way you have planned. In the midst of change happening all around you, acceptance means recognizing the possibilities of what might happen at some point. Considering what you would do with yourself in even the worst conditions is how you prepare for anything while letting go of your need for something specific.

Technique: The Life You Don't Expect

Turn to a blank page in your journal and at the top of the page, write "What I will do if..." Finish the sentence by writing in something you don't want to happen. For example, your sentence might say, "What I will do if I end up alone." On the line below your statement, begin writing how you will handle the situation that the line you wrote describes.

This may take some time to think of what to write. Many of us have never considered the possibility of life happening completely differently than we anticipate. But acknowledging how you might address such "worst-case scenarios" will help you prepare for not getting what you want out of life and moving on from it. It is the moments in which you know you will be okay no matter what happens that you are most easily able to accept what comes your way.

———

Give yourself breathing room from your fear. When you prepare yourself for anything, you know you can handle anything. You no longer worry as much. But something else happens when you feel prepared. You stop emphasizing the importance of the past, what may come about in the future, and immediate problems you encounter. Basically, you stop putting an emphasis on results. Instead, you believe in yourself—something that is likely long overdue.

When you feel prepared and are accepting of life, a great deal of your emotional distress dissipates; and in a way, this may feel as though you are losing the intensity from your life. The truth is that you will probably lose some of your intensity, but when change happens, you always lose a part of yourself. In the passage of one moment to the next, we are always leaving behind parts of our lives while gaining something new. It's the exchange of energy, like the cycle of our breaths, in which we must let go of what is gone and welcome what exists. Both involve acceptance.

The two words that arouse the strongest emotions are "hello" and "goodbye." And as you say hello to a life without depression, you must say goodbye to the intensity that comes with extremism. Good times won't feel as amazing as they once did as an extremist, but bad times also won't leave you devastated and determined to fight for what you want. The highs of an extremist mentality are incredible. I know this, but I also know that the lows can bring your entire life to a halt.

This world is constantly turning, exposing us to night and day. And embracing this world means accepting that some moments will be darker than others. But standing in one spot, demanding that your way is the only way means there is no room for growth; it means there is no room for calmness. Living without depression, however, means being able to be at peace with yourself.

Calmness creates silence in your life. And while you may not want silence right now—possibly correlating it with emptiness, numbness, or loneliness—what the silence of calmness gives you is a break from your worry. It allows you to relax and breathe easy. When you think about calmness this way, it might not seem so bad. Happiness doesn't always mean you are smiling; it can just as well mean being content.

Not every thing means everything.

Chapter 13

Judge Not, Lest Ye Be Judged

There are two ways to change your life: change the world or change your relationship to the world. Trying to change the world is a lot more difficult than changing yourself, and you'll succeed much less. Truthfully, even if you were able to change the world, your relationship to it would change soon after. Just as all things change at some point, you must make necessary changes to yourself when it is time. And depression is a signal that the time has come to make those changes to your life.

Too often people don't look to themselves to make change; they look to others. They hold opinions about the way the world should be and get upset when it doesn't conform to those opinions. They see injustice around them, and many times they begin treating the world with disregard because they don't feel like they can make a difference. In essence, they just stop caring.

Of course, not caring is not the answer because a lack of care is exactly what you feel in depression. Since you are a part of this world, the way you treat your surroundings extends to the way you treat yourself. So any lack of care you may have about this world affects your concern for your own life. You end up feeling lonely, unimportant, and hurt.

There is an age-old question that asks why bad things happen to good people, but there are two major flaws in asking a question like this. The first is the assumption that certain experiences are strictly bad and that the people experiencing them are purely good. As discussed already, no one thing is entirely good or bad. However, when you view a situation as exclusively negative, you fail to see ways in which you can benefit from the situation. You also create hostility in your life as it often becomes impossible for anyone to convince you of potential opportunities within your circumstances. Anyone trying to convince you of a positive perspective seems wrong and ignorant of what you are going through. So your circumstances make you depressed while your stubbornness that there is no other way to view your situation locks you into that depression. You embrace the pain of the experience, stuck in a perspective of negativity.

The second flaw in the question of why bad things happen to good people is the suggestion that good people deserve good things. The truth of the matter is that no one deserves anything specific in this world. When you feel like you deserve something, replace the word "deserve" with the word "want." Then you can decide whether you are getting enough from situations for what you are putting into them.

If you believe your character entitles you to good things, whenever you encounter troubles, you will take them personally. Interestingly, feelings of entitlement and elitism typically come from a lack of self-esteem because you are depending on the outside world to display confirmation of your self-worth. The problem, of course, is that if your experiences are not in line with what you believe you deserve, you are left without any cause to feel good.

By stubbornly believing that your life is not the way it was meant to be, you maintain an egotistical perspective, only caring about your view of the world. However, when you're depressed, you also give up on yourself. This is doubly damaging: self-centered on the outside coupled with self-disregard on the inside. By believing that you deserve certain pleasures while simultaneously not caring about your life, you create an internal struggle in which you only want what you don't have but don't care when you get it. Can you think of a way in which you can be happy living like this? I can't. You're constantly unsatisfied, searching for more, and feeling like your life is doomed.

In this world, you often get out what you put in. But if you wait around for the world to give you what you want or to treat you some particular way, you may end up waiting a long time. If you want something, make an effort to bring it into your life. This book has consistently discussed how effort is related to control and how what you do makes you who you are, but if you don't think you are accurately being identified by the way you are living, then you are judging yourself based on results.

Judging Yourself

You may have been told that you were special at some point in your life. Or you may have instead been told that you were not good enough to make something of yourself. Neither of these is true. This is important to understand as characterizing people as "special" or "not good enough" suggests that they are different from everyone else. They then have to live up to or overcome some standard as opposed to just being okay with who they are.

Too often those people who grew up hearing that they were special put pressure on themselves to live up to that perception. Their approval of themselves is based upon setting themselves apart from others to maintain that level of "special." They, therefore, define excellence not just by doing well but by doing better than others. It's not just enough to win; everyone else must lose. They think there is no excuse for not being the best.

Conversely, those who grew up hearing that they were not good enough may believe that every failing is the fault of who they are. Because they see themselves as inferior to others, they interpret another's success as confirmation of their own failures in life. They then often give up trying to improve their lives, believing that who they are is an excuse for not achieving excellence.

What many people don't understand in raising children is that while everyone wants to be important, everyone really just wants to be accepted. Each of us just wants to know that we are good enough the way we are rather than being told that we are something other than normal. It doesn't mean there isn't room for improvement; it just means that there is nothing wrong with who we are as human beings. When you're convinced that you are better or worse than others, every failure intensifies your insecurities that you're not good enough.

The truth is you are not better or worse than anyone else. Talent comes from practice; judgments are never unanimous, and hard work doesn't guarantee the results you want. You are as capable as you are determined to be capable, and you determine your own self-worth by following through on what is important to you.

Just as you must not allow others' critiques of you to determine your value, you must not allow others' experiences to serve as a gauge to measure your self-worth either. You may have intelligence, charisma, good looks, a sense of humor, or a host of other great qualities; but your life is based solely on what you do with it, not what characteristics others have used to gain prosperity. You may have failed out of school, had a drug addiction, lied to people, been to prison, attempted suicide, been homeless, or experienced a variety of misfortunes that have ruined others' lives; but that doesn't have to determine your life. You have to let go of the past and the resulting present by not using the word "should"—"How you think your life *should* be" or "What you think you *should* have gotten."

What matters is not where you come from or what you receive but what you do with your life. Looking outside yourself at others, believing that someone else has advantages that you don't or that it's unfair that your life is more difficult than another's only takes your focus off what's truly important: who you are, what you have, and what you do with each.

Jealousy

When you hold a specific perspective about what is deserved and what isn't, you can end up believing that some people do not deserve the advantages they receive. It's the opposite of questioning why bad things happen to good people; it is questioning why good things happen to bad people. The same flaws exist in this debate, however, because of the misconceptions of justice and that people and experiences are either strictly good or bad.

By focusing on what you believe other people deserve while simultaneously having a negative perspective of your own life, your focus can quickly turn to jealousy. You disregard everything you have and yearn for what others have. But you are not judging others when you are jealous; you are judging yourself. You are saying that what you have isn't enough. And you know what? That's true because what you have won't make you happy unless you are doing something with it worth appreciating.

When you are jealous of others, you value what you don't have rather than what you do have; and the reason you think this way is probably because you're not doing much with what you do have. And here, we come right back around to effort once again. Until you start making the most of what you have instead of expecting results to forever make you happy, what you have will never be enough.

The negativity that exists in jealousy can consume your overall outlook on life as you not only see yourself as without the successes that others enjoy but feel like others should not have those pleasures. You think that good experiences bestowed upon other people, particularly those you don't like, make your life harder. You look down on the world and yourself, feeling as though everyone else has talent, advantages, and pleasures that you don't (even though you have just as much potential as anyone). You relinquish control of your own happiness to the experiences in others' lives.

Well, it's time to stop focusing on what you didn't get or what you think anyone deserves. When you find yourself jealous of someone else, think about what you have and what you could do with it. Once you start making the most of what you have, you start appreciating it. Once you start appreciating what you have, you won't get stuck lamenting what you don't have. Once you stop feeling bad about what you don't have, you start feeling good for what other people have because when you appreciate your own life, you become equally happy for others' well-being. You surround yourself with positive energy rather than self-loathing and envy.

Judging the World around You

When you judge yourself, you judge everyone. By judging how you believe you deserve to be treated, you naturally judge people by how they treat you. However, judgment of others typically occurs even when the relationship between you and those people is loosely connected because you feel that what they are doing impacts your life in some way. But the concern about how you will be impacted is commonly due to a lack of understanding.

Negative judgments are often related to behaviors and activities with which we have no prior experience. We only know the experiences we have had and, therefore, unfamiliar activities in which other people engage may sometimes appear strange and inappropriate. Without understanding the behavior of others, many people occasionally fear that others' actions could affect their own lives significantly. They may overestimate the significance of what they don't understand. And because of the meaning they attribute to other people's behavior, they doubt their own ability to handle it and worry about what will happen if they can't handle it. And with feelings of doubt and worry festering, they are unable to be happy.

This is a major reason why so many people fear cultures that are different from their own. Some see others celebrating a different religion as a belittlement of their own religion. Some see others enjoying a different lifestyle as an encroachment upon their own lifestyle. And many of us even judge the actions of those we love because we fear what they are doing will threaten our relationships with them. But just because you are unfamiliar with another way of living doesn't mean your comfort is in jeopardy because of it.

Another reason why many of us judge others is because of low self-esteem. When you judge someone negatively, you believe that you do what is right and that person doesn't. You create a comparison in which you can raise yourself above the person since you are the one setting the standards with which you judge.

While placing yourself above someone can make you feel better, the feeling is only temporary. It only lasts until that person is gone and you no longer have someone to compare yourself to. This can often cause people to end up judging others throughout their lives to consistently create comparisons with those they encounter and get back that feeling of superiority.

When you make comparisons between you and other people, you stop basing your happiness on how well you are living up to your principles. You instead look at how poorly others are living up to your principles. But judging people negatively on how you believe they should be acting doesn't say anything about how well you are honoring your principles. Regardless of how anybody else in this world acts, to be the person you want to be, *you* have to follow through on actions that honor that lifestyle.

The late comedian George Carlin once said, "Have you ever noticed when you're driving that anyone who's driving slower than you is an idiot, and anyone driving faster than you is a maniac?"[1] No one is virtuous and skilled all the time, yet many believe that they should be free to criticize another for what they believe they would do if they were in that person's situation. However, because they are not in the situation at the time they are making their criticism, they feel justified in their view. Then when they end up in similar circumstances, they are almost always prepared with an excuse for why their own actions are different from those of someone whom they previously judged.

It is essential that you consider whether you live by a double standard in which you are always right and others are wrong for the same things. Don't let what others do bother you while committing similar actions when in similar circumstances. It's much easier to judge than to look within at how you might act were you in the same situation. Everyone makes mistakes, and everyone handles life differently.

Judging people based on their actions is not entirely bad. It's the only way to form opinions that help you determine what to bring in or remove from your life. What you want to avoid is judging people solely on one of many actions. As discussed in the chapter on hope, it's important to understand what intentions existed behind someone's actions. Since effort does not always lead to the intended results, being quick to judge someone can cause negative feelings without good reason. It will, therefore, be your job to explore an isolated act before using it as a gauge to judge an entire person.

There will, however, be many situations in your life when you do not have the time, ability, or desire to investigate someone's intentions. Particularly when you will not be making an effort to uncover the root of an action, it is all the more important to avoid judging someone. This is because quickly judging people can cause *you* personal grief. If you become someone who is quick to judge others, believing that your way is always the right way, you will end up believing that everyone else does things incorrectly. Your seemingly harmless criticism of others in this world will build up your perspective that the world is filled with people creating problems for you.

Being quick to judge others allows you to convince yourself that the problems in your own life are the result of unavoidable problems in this world. You give yourself reasons to avoid working on improving your own life while cursing the world in which you live. This is the perspective of someone stuck in a rut of depression, feeling incapable of making change.

I admit that it's easy to get frustrated with others, particularly those you don't know. Cursing other drivers while stuck in traffic, belittling customer service agents over the phone, or yelling about politicians are common daily practices for many people. But every time you look down on someone else, you end up bringing a little bit of negativity into your life. You throw your energy away in a useless act of condemnation. And over time, those insignificant displays of negativity add up to a significant feeling of negativity until you feel as though you are stuck in a world in which you are constantly fighting to get by.

Technique: It's Okay

In order to stop judging people, you must accept their flaws. You need to realize that no one and nothing is perfect and that you will encounter things you don't like throughout your life. And just as you want the opportunity to live your life as you see fit, you must also be willing to allow other people to live their own lives as they choose.

Stopping yourself from quickly judging others does not mean you have to like what they are doing. You don't have to agree with it, but to be able to avoid letting its occurrence disrupt your life, you must learn to be okay with it. So say, "Okay."

As you encounter situations you don't like and are not truly life-altering, say "Okay" out loud. If you are driving and someone cuts you off but doesn't harm you, say "Okay." If you're talking on a cell phone and the call is dropped, say "Okay." Even if you say "okay" in a sarcastic tone, you will still hear yourself accepting the situation. So rather than getting frustrated with a temporary experience, admit your acceptance of what has happened; and see where it takes you.

Why the Golden Rule Matters

Nearly everyone has heard of the Golden Rule, which says, "Do unto others as you would have them do unto you." This is an important concept, but like many pieces of advice, it can be misinterpreted either in how it should be put into action or its reasoning as to why it is important. In the case of the Golden Rule, people typically look at how they are treated and respond similarly while some follow the credo more accurately by treating others the way they would like to be treated. But there is a meaning more substantial to the Golden Rule that often gets overlooked. It involves perspective. It is my belief that the true, and often unrealized, meaning behind the

Golden Rule is that *the way you view others is how you believe others view you.*

You are not in anyone else's head but your own. And so without the knowledge of how different people view you, you are left only with your own perspective of yourself as a means of determining how those you encounter look at you.

It's only natural to think that others see in you what you see in yourself. However, your view of yourself is not just in line with how you believe other people see you; your view of yourself is also in line with how you look at others.

When you view people in a certain light, whatever you focus on most will stand out to you. Similarly, when you look at yourself, those same things that you focus on in others will stand out to you. For example, if you typically focus on the mistakes that other people make, you will very likely also be critical of yourself when you screw up because mistakes hold a great deal of significance for you regardless of who makes those mistakes. When you then interpret how others view you, you will believe that your mistakes stand out to them because they are what stand out to you.

The truth is that people do not always see this world in the same way, but the way you view others is often identical to your interpretation of the way they view you even if they don't actually see you that way. This means that by changing the way you view the people around you, you can effectively change the way you believe those people view you. If you focus on the good in others and accept their flaws, you will soon feel like others similarly appreciate what you do well and accept you regardless of your own shortcomings.

By giving less significance to any characteristic that you see in the world around you, you stop being as concerned with how anyone views that same characteristic in yourself because it no longer holds as much value to you. You end up getting out of your relationships exactly what you put in or don't put in. Changing your perspective of others to change your interpretation of their perspective of you removes both your own insecurities as well as helps you appreciate all the world has to offer rather than judging that it should somehow be different.

The Golden Rule is understood to be about treatment, but consider that the way you view others is how you treat them mentally. People often focus on physical treatment more than emotional treatment because it is out in the open, but as I have mentioned, it is the intentions behind actions that matter. Your perspective is actually more important than your physical action because your view of the world doesn't just guide how you act physically; it also affects how you interpret your experiences.

How You Change the World

While acceptance of the world is fundamental to moving on with your life, you may believe that there are some problems in this world that are inherently wrong and must be resolved. You may believe that some people are doing the wrong things and must be stopped—even if that means using force. While force is a viable way to change others, without constant monitoring, people will rebel, break their silence, and return to their original ways because force doesn't change people's beliefs; inspiration does.

Whether you grew up believing that you would one day change the world or never thought your life would amount to much, many people only end up criticizing what happens in the world. They want the world to be different, but they do nothing to improve it, having thoughts like, "What can I do?" As you must know by now, the only way to get anything accomplished in this world is to make an effort, and your effort is something that represents who you are. So it should come as no surprise that the way you truly have an impact on the world, which you may be judging negatively, is to lead by example.

No one has ever "changed the world" without help. Every great leader memorialized in history books made a difference in this world by influencing those he/she encountered through the way he/she lived, and over time, the people who that person influenced changed the world in some way. It was the masses that chose to follow the lead of the ones who inspired them.

People have to make their own choices. The world will follow you if it chooses, but if you choose first how the world should be, you're misunderstanding the way the world works. You are not here to change the world, nor are you here to let it change you. You are here to be a part of this world, acting and reacting, doing what is right, and being proud of the life you choose to live. And when you live like this, you just might make the world a better place.

The idea that your life or the world around you should be any particular way locks you into a series of judgments that not even you can live up to. Everything will change, but instead of instinctively judging, ask yourself why you believe things should be different than they are. The purpose of judgment is for you to determine how to live your own life. Sometimes your judgments have value, such as when you are in a situation that is repeatedly making you feel bad. And when you make a decision to improve your life based on your judgment of the situation, judgment serves its purpose.

Too often though, judgment rises from a failure to appreciate what you have, a lack of understanding, or low self-esteem. And with any of these at the root of your judgment, you will only see what's wrong in the world. You will grow jealous, critical, and fearful that others are looking down on you. And when you become someone who is quick to judge, you give up your opportunity for acceptance, understanding, and growth—all because you want to be right.

One thing you have in common with the people
around you is that you all ended up in the same place.

Chapter 14

The World Doesn't Revolve around You

You are not alone. There is a great deal of comfort in knowing that other people feel the way you do, particularly when you don't feel happy. It's hard enough to feel sad in life, but it's even harder when you think you're the only one who feels that way. However, I assure you, that's never the case. There are people throughout this world who feel how you feel, and each of them has a choice with what to do with those feelings.

The idea that we have something in common with other people is what bonds us to them. So often those who experience difficult situations together feel themselves more united by being able to lean on each other and because they can relate through the shared experience. Most of the time, however, our challenges are not shared experiences. And so we don't feel those connections with others. We see our hardships as unique to us. We focus almost exclusively on ourselves and create separation between us and everyone else.

We give up this opportunity for comfort not because we don't want the connection with others but because we don't see the connection. When we look at the world, we always experience it through our own eyes. Based on what *we* know, what *we've* been through, and what *we* have, *we* interpret the world by our own perspectives. And so without someone else going through an experience with us, it's hard to imagine that anyone else knows how we are feeling.

Our views about this world are shaped by a number of different sources from our past experiences to our current moods, but one thing that often guides our perspectives about situations is how we believe those situations affect us. We typically interpret what is good and bad based upon whether we get what we want. Many of us make judgments about others because of what we believe their actions imply about their feelings toward us. And sometimes we even determine if we are doing what is right with our own lives by what we encounter with others.

Focusing on your own life and how you are affected by the world around you is essential. It is all part of discovering patterns and making decisions about what to do with your life, but what is also essential is understanding that what you encounter is not always related to you. People make decisions and events transpire all the time that have nothing to do with you. Just because you may feel an effect by what you encounter doesn't mean it was intentional or inappropriate. If you take everything personally, everything you witness that you disagree with will feel like a personal attack. And eventually, you'll end up turning against everyone.

It's a difficult proposition to focus on your relationships with everyone and everything around you while simultaneously knowing that what others do is not always linked to your life. But the fact is that while the world does not revolve around you, your experience of the world revolves around your perception of it.

It's Not Always Personal

The idea that "the world doesn't revolve around you" is often thought of in a selfish manner in that you will not always get what you want. However, there is another side to it (a good side); it is the fact that the things people do that affect you are not always personal. This is important to know because many times when you interpret a person's actions or comments to mean something negative about you, it's not always the case. For example, if a person questions whether you are prepared to take on a specific challenge and you take the question personally, it may seem like the person doubts your abilities. However, this negative experience might all occur in your mind without that person ever saying he/she doesn't believe in you.

We are the ones who create the connections between what we encounter and what we feel. Many of us see outside sources as the reasons for why we often feel the way we do, but the actions of others only affect you as much as you let them. Take the time to really consider what people say and do and if they might actually be curious, helpful, or joking around. Too often another's inquisitiveness, advice, or sarcasm is taken the wrong way.

When it comes to your interactions with others in which you get upset, your mood is often a reason. For example, if you are already upset and someone makes a joke about you, you might be more prone to getting mad at the person than laughing it off. However, when you are depressed about your life, your underlying negative feelings are constantly present and playing a role in how you interpret the world around you.

With depression, you are unfulfilled in this world; you are disappointed with yourself, and you are uncertain about your direction in life. So when anyone says or does something that could be taken to mean that he/she doesn't like you or that you are doing something wrong with your life, it's easy to take it personally. You get upset because of your fear that the person's comments, questions, or actions confirm your own negative thoughts about yourself.

We often respond to this perceived confirmation of negativity with more negativity. We become defensive in order to push away what feels like an attack from someone else. Sometimes we go so far as to convince ourselves that we don't like someone in order to disregard the value of that person's opinion. So we prove the person wrong not by criticizing the criticism but by criticizing the criticizer.

In my own life, I recall during the writing of this book that I once set a goal to finish writing it by my birthday. I told a friend that it would be my birthday present to myself. My friend responded by saying, "You are writing a self-help book for yourself? What does that say about you?" I immediately and instinctively interpreted that my friend questioning my actions meant there must be something wrong with what I was doing. I initially became angry and was about to comment on something my friend had done wrong to even the playing field, but then I realized what kind of person it made me to write a self-help book in part for myself. It made me the type of person that treats others who need help with the same respect I needed to give myself when I needed help. We do treat the world like we treat ourselves, and that was what I needed to explain to my friend. But more importantly, it was what I needed to realize for myself because what self-help really means is helping yourself. Once I looked past my own insecurity about what my friend was saying, I realized that there wasn't anything wrong in what I was doing. Suddenly, my friend's curiosity was no longer a condemnation of me but just a question.

When you have depression or are even depressed about a particular experience, you seemingly live your life on the defensive, ready to pounce on anyone who you believe is implying you're not doing what you should be doing with yourself. Even when it comes to the advice you get, with depression you walk a fine line between looking for the right answers and rejecting anyone else telling you how to live your life. Deep down, we all want to constantly be moving in a direction of betterment; but many of us tend to look at anything that contradicts what we are doing as an insinuation that we're not moving in a positive direction. However, the reality is that when it comes to the things people say to you or about you that strike a nerve, that nerve is almost always your own insecurity.

Rather than reacting defensively on instinct, evaluate your feelings and understand them. You may have good reason to be upset about what someone has said or done, but you may also just be blowing it out of proportion. It may actually be your own hostile reactions to misinterpretations that cause people to begin negatively judging you. What do you really think would happen if you just let go of some of the negativity you encounter?

Taking the actions of others personally does not just relate to negativity; it can involve good feelings too. Consider someone doing something nice for you. If you mistake the possibility that the person is simply being nice, you may believe the person is acting that way specifically because of you. Your misinterpretation could lead to having affectionate feelings for someone that are not mutual. You then set yourself up for rejection simply because you disregarded the possibility that the person's personality wasn't influenced by you.

Intentions are not always clear, and in order to know what someone's actions mean, you simply have to ask. Your inquisitiveness may be an extra step in determining how to respond, but it can significantly shorten the duration and intensity of any experience by getting out the truth about what is fueling someone's behavior. While people will not always know how to respond to your inquisitiveness, in time you may find that your decision not to take an experience personally but to instead open up the lines of communication can create that connection I spoke of at the beginning of the chapter.

While it is true that sometimes a person's mannerisms provide good indications about how he/she feels about you, there are more factors guiding people's actions than just you. As your relationships develop, you will come to learn more about the typical characteristics of the people with whom you share those relationships and what their actions imply. However, if you always assume what another's actions mean and never inquire as to the different possible reasons behind those actions, your relationships will dissolve.

Not Getting What You Want

In addition to the positive side of the world not revolving around you, there is also the consequence of you not always getting what you want in life. It's the opposite of when interactions that you don't like take place; it's when interactions that you want or expect *don't* take place. While not always the case, these two opposites typically occur in tandem. For example, you might get upset when people don't do certain things and simultaneously want them to be doing something different. Or when people do things you don't want them to do, they're not always doing what you want them to do.

The fact is that you don't always get what you want. This is something you surely realize as having depression is filled with experiences in which you don't get what you desire. However, when you focus on what *you* don't get, you again destroy the possibility of connection between you and other people. The truth is that you have your own life to lead, and you are truly free to lead your life in any way you choose regardless of what you may always think. But what you must also recognize is that everyone else has that same right as you. And it is *that* sameness in which the connection between you and other people exists.

As I spoke about in the last chapter, there is nothing that we deserve in life. It is up to each of us to go after what we seek, but if we disregard the desires of others, we just create more separation. Let's say, for example, that you weren't invited to a party. If you disregard the right of the person to invite whomever he/she wants, all you will focus on is what you want. More specifically, you will focus on how you didn't get what you want because of that person. You create a rift in your relationship with that person. Now you may believe that the separation between you and the other person was caused by him/her only thinking about him/herself and not inviting you, but the separation you feel is caused by *your* opinion of the way things should be.

It is my personal belief that one of the most painful challenges in life to overcome is the feeling of rejection. The idea that you are not wanted can wreak havoc on your self-esteem. You end up pushing away a world that you think doesn't want you. The truth, however, is that you have a role to play in this world; but you don't have a role to play in every part of this world. And would you really want that? For so many people, the reason they feel exhausted in life is because they try to be a part of everything. But the more you have in your life, the more things there are that require your attention. You can't be everywhere. You can't do everything. Let go of the need to be involved all the time.

Instead of expecting that other people should always consider your feelings, consider whether your feelings really need to be a factor in another's decisions. How involved are you in a particular situation that warrants your feelings being taken into account? Just as you don't base your decisions around everyone and everything in this world, neither does anyone else.

There are countless reasons that things do and do not happen in this world, but sometimes we give circumstances meaning that just isn't there. In fact, the reason we often suspect that others don't do the things we want is typically the same reason that we suspect people do the things we don't want. And while we typically cite others' personalities as the reason behind their decisions, deep down we fear that *we* are the reason.

Feeling as though people owe you things in this world will only make you frustrated every time someone doesn't live up to your expectations. You may not always agree with what other people choose to do with their lives, but that's not your decision; it's theirs. Your decision is how to respond. And if you want something in life, *you* have to go after it.

Sitting on the sidelines of this world, complaining about what you didn't get will never fulfill you. Stop looking to the world to give to you and start putting forth effort toward getting what you want. Life is about participation. It's an interactive world, not just a visual one.

Sometimes simply asking for what you want is enough. Sometimes getting what you want requires more effort than that. And sometimes, no matter how hard you work, you still won't get what you want. But it's up to you to make yourself feel involved in this world.

Most people are waiting for others to ask them to participate, but your invitation to this world is your life. The day you were born, you were given an opportunity to do whatever you wanted in this world. And every day you are alive, you have that same opportunity. It's time to RSVP to that invitation to this world and get the type of life you want regardless of what others do or don't do.

Giving Up Your Life for Others

You are affected by everything you encounter in this world, but it doesn't always mean that the circumstances surrounding each encounter exist because of you. When you take your encounters personally, you are judging what the actions of others mean about you. And when you judge the actions of others, you likewise think that your actions are being judged. This can cause you to overthink your own decisions and worry that you've done the wrong things in life.

If your actions are tied to the views of others, you spend your life being concerned about how you are viewed. While monitoring your behavior so as to create good relationships with the people around you is important, by having an abundance of focus on what others think of you, you have a lack of focus on what you think of yourself. You disregard what makes you genuine in the hope of winning the approval of others.

When you live a life in which you believe everything you do is being judged, you give up your greatest strength. You are unable to be yourself. You end up living your life in fear, concerned that you might say or do the wrong thing. You might clam up, unwilling to share your true feelings because of how you will be perceived. You may even worry that being nice to one person will make others feel unloved. You concentrate so hard on trying to interpret others' feelings that you forget the importance of interpreting your own.

There is no doubt that what you do has an effect on others and a significant effect on your own perception of yourself, but one action isn't everything. You can't spend your life worrying that the people around you will take everything you do personally. The fact is people aren't always thinking about you, and they aren't always judging you. The world just doesn't revolve around you.

Your life is only yours to live, and the best step you can take toward creating a life in which you are not concerned about others taking your actions personally is to not take *their* actions personally. It's really just one in the same; not taking others' actions personally just means not worrying about how they feel about you. And when you give up your worry, the significance of their judgment fades and you can be yourself without hesitation.

Don't Take Life So Seriously

Look around you. Read the news. Turn on the television. All over are people criticizing, protesting, and arguing about the decisions, actions, and lifestyles of others. For so many people, every issue seems like a battle. The amount of hatred and animosity in this world boils down to people feeling like others are imposing on their right to be happy—but there is no happiness in fighting.

In an effort to stop the shouting in your head, you must give up the war. Realize that others aren't always against you and their actions aren't necessarily disenfranchising you. You are free to be you, but when you fight, you're not free because what you're fighting for *is* the freedom to be you.

Too often we take life too seriously. And when we take our lives so seriously, we tend to take everything that we experience very personally. We see the actions of others and feel like they infringe on our own lives. But everyone wants freedom. Everyone wants happiness. This world is filled with opportunities to play, be silly, and joke around; but so many people miss out on this. Those who shout from the mountaintops to fight over every issue are missing the point of what they are fighting for.

There is no question that some issues in life are serious and worth standing up for, but take a moment and consider the following: *What in your life isn't worth fighting over?* In an effort to stop taking everything so personally, you have to stop taking life so seriously.

Use this moment right now to take a slow deep breath, in and out. Breathe out the demands, the fears, and the intensity. Do this and suddenly you become free again. Life does not need to be so serious. This world needs more joy, not more aggression. Your life needs more joy, not more aggression. In this world, you won't always get what you want or be treated the way you think is right; but that doesn't always mean your life is worse off because of it. While we all want everything to be exactly the way we believe it should be, what you probably need more right now is simply to relax.

In order to feel like you are a part of this world, you must feel a connection with everyone around you. But when you focus exclusively on yourself, you lose sight of everyone else that exists; and the opportunity for that connection disappears. Only once you recognize the importance of others to live their own lives for themselves along with the importance for you to live your life for yourself will you begin to create a connection between you and the world around you. You begin to see that we are all just trying to be happy. We all experience episodes of fear, doubt, and loneliness. And we all have the opportunity to do great things that make us proud of ourselves.

We are all in this world together. And together we can improve our lives; we just can't be dependent on each other to determine our own worth. What people say and do in this world is not always a commentary on your lifestyle. And at the same time, what people say and do doesn't require your approval. But when you take the time to stop and think about other people's needs, consider how they might be feeling, and reach out your hand to them, your own fears, doubts, and loneliness vanish because together you share an experience.

You are the reason you feel the way you feel.

Chapter 15

The Two Sides of Help

I mentioned early on in this book that the transfer of energy that must occur in your life is about getting and giving. This exchange extends to all areas of your life as you interact with this world every day. So naturally, the two sides of help that affect your view of life are receiving and providing it.

Many people are almost instinctively opposed to asking for or accepting help as well as providing help to others. The avoidance of help, however, makes it difficult to avoid depression because both getting and giving help are related to how you feel about your own importance in this world. Getting help proves that others care about you and giving help lets you realize that other people need you.

Asking for Help

One of the hardest tasks for many people is asking for help. Too often many of us assume that asking another person for help is a confession of weakness or failure. We feel embarrassed and believe that asking for help shows we are incapable of accomplishing a goal on our own. Other times, we simply don't want to bother people with our problems, believing we should be able to handle them on our own. And sometimes we avoid asking for help because we don't believe anyone else is capable of getting things done the way we want.

Asking for help, however, is proof that you are determined to succeed and are wise enough to use all the resources in your life to make that happen. The people around you are there for reasons, and like everything in your life, you should make the most of them. Asking for help opens up a new method for success and provides you something you desperately need: proof that others care about you. While you may not always get assistance from the specific people you want help from, you should be less focused on them and more focused on getting the help you need. There are friends, family members, organizations, and many others that you might not normally turn to who may be ready and willing to help you out.

When you refuse to ask for help from others, you make tasks more difficult than they need to be by closing yourself off from the world. You prohibit people who might want to help you from proving how much they care about you. Have you ever considered that the reason you may feel like your life is filled with difficulties or that no one cares about your well-being is because you never stopped and asked others for help?

It is not always easy to ask for help because it involves admitting that you're not perfect. It means putting aside your fears of judgment and being confident enough to ask for a hand. I realize that many people do not always have this confidence in themselves, but I also know that there are always people around who want to help. People like to feel useful. It's the reason it seems that others often want to give advice. So if you need help and others may want to help, this makes for a good exchange.

It's important for you to realize that your refusal to ask for help or even accept help may be closely related to how you view your own effort. If you usually turn a cold shoulder to the support others offer you, you very well may be similarly disregarding all the help you provide yourself. That means that even when you work hard to accomplish something completely on your own, you probably don't even give yourself credit for it. And without acknowledgement for what you do, your effort won't ever give you a feeling of pride in yourself. You'll simply feel like you're constantly working without ever really accomplishing anything of value.

Utilizing the help of others can make a significant difference in your life, but that doesn't mean you always need to accept others' help because a life without your own effort is a life without meaning. Even when you do accept help from others, it will still be important that you make an effort to help yourself because you also need proof that *you* care about yourself. And when you put forth your own effort, the feeling you get from accomplishment is that much more rewarding because of the role you played in it.

When you work for something and others help you, you also create a bond with them. When you ask someone else for help, it tells that person that you believe in his/her ability to help you. This vote of confidence can make another person feel really good. So you end up giving someone a good feeling by asking for help, and you get a good feeling by learning that you can depend on that person—all the while easing some of the load required in what you are working toward. What could have originally been a challenging task suddenly becomes mutually beneficial. You both help each other and consequently strengthen your relationship.

For many of us, we strive to be independent by taking on every challenge on our own; but we'd be so much better off if we just asked for help. Doing something nice based on your needs is the only way for someone to show you that he/she cares about your welfare. But by inhibiting others from helping you, you eventually interpret those in your life (including yourself) as not caring for you. And that's a pretty good reason to feel depressed.

Helping Others

Effort is key. If you completely rely on others to provide for you, you'll never learn how to rely on yourself. Part of your effort, however, needs to include giving help to other people. For the same reasons that made it beneficial for another person to help you out, giving help can prove to you how much others need you in their lives. You also can improve your relationships with them by showing your consideration and reliability.

When suffering from depression, you often have personal doubts about your own importance in the world. By helping others, you become an important part of their lives. As I mentioned in Chapter 13, the most effective way to change the world is to set an example for others to follow. When you give, you set that example. You set the bar high, and when others see your benevolence, they are likely to be appreciative and similarly help others.

Do not always expect that by helping out a particular person that he/she will return the favor to you. In many cases, this will happen. However, sometimes your kindness will encourage the person to help out someone else who needs help. In this way, not only have you helped someone out; but you started a chain of events that is bringing more kindness to this world. While you may never fully know the impact of your actions, I promise you that your interactions with others have a significant effect on their attitudes toward life. The purpose of you giving help to another is to make a difference, and if you acknowledge that, the feeling you get from helping someone is more valuable than any favor you could ask for in return.

Technique: Volunteering

One of the best ways to help others in need is to volunteer your time and energy. Donating money to a foundation is simply not enough. In order to really help others and help yourself in the process, you'll have to contribute some form of help that involves your own effort. It might mean giving up an entire day of your weekend, but that's the point of volunteering. It means standing up for something besides yourself, and the impact you will have on others and yourself will likely make it an activity that ends up on the "<u>YES</u>" side of your "After the Fact" lists.

Volunteer to work at homeless shelters, animal shelters, churches, synagogues, hospitals, the Red Cross, Habitat for Humanity, Easter Seals, or any other charitable organization. You can even look up <u>www.VolunteerMatch.org</u> online, which currently lists volunteer opportunities throughout the United

States. Where and how you volunteer is up to you. What matters is that you contribute your time and energy to a charitable cause. You may just realize how much you have taken for granted in your life as you become a first-hand witness to those who are worse off than you and how fortunate your life really is.

———

Beyond volunteering, you can make a difference with people you encounter on a daily basis by helping them feel better about their lives. I remember once being at a costume party and seeing a couple walking side by side with each other. I stopped them and told them that they both looked great. They then turned and complimented each other on how great each looked. I realized that neither person in this couple had acknowledged the effort the other had put into dressing up. They then turned around and walked away together. Metaphorically, I felt like they were walking in a new direction with their relationship for the moment; but one thing I knew for sure was that I helped make their night a better one. That story and the feeling of making a difference remain with me to this day, and all I did was compliment two people I didn't even know.

Help can come in several different forms. It may be a favor to make life easier, a few words of encouragement, or just a compliment to make someone smile. But as I mentioned, it's important for each of us to help ourselves. There is an old proverb that says, "Give a man a fish and you feed him for a day. Teach a man to fish and you feed him for a lifetime."[1] The idea behind this is that it is better to help others to help themselves than to just do something for them. Even the people I complimented used that opportunity to help their relationship with each other. It's when you help in this way that you have a lasting effect on others because the knowledge and confidence they gain by counting on themselves will remain with them whereas you will not. So when you help others, make your help a byproduct of teamwork. Everyone will appreciate the effort that much more than being the lone person giving or getting.

An inevitable consequence of helping people to help themselves is that those people you help won't always help themselves. Your assistance won't always make a big difference in others' lives because you can't make people help themselves if they don't want to. Just as you are the one who must get yourself through this life, others must do the same for themselves. Don't take their decisions too personally. Remember, your effort is more important than the results you witness. And while you won't motivate everyone you set out to help, it doesn't mean you shouldn't try.

In a world where it takes effort to feel good, encourage, encourage, encourage. Don't be a naysayer, dissuading others from pursuing their dreams. Give them the push they need to make an effort. It's what I'm doing for you right now in this book. You never know exactly what your effort might lead to in the future, and someone just might thank you in the most gracious of ways someday.

There are opportunities every day to help others. Keep your eyes open for them. Giving someone who is stranded a lift, letting someone who seems to be in a hurry get in front of you in line, or offering your leftovers to someone who is homeless are just a few examples. Sometimes just giving a little can mean a lot to others, and sometimes it can feel like a lot to you too. Many of us, however, give up opportunities to help those who need it for three reasons: fear, laziness, or selfishness.

In terms of fear, modern-day news has spent years convincing the public that they are in constant danger. Headlines detail the rare events when people are murdered, swindled out of money, or injured when trusting others. This publicity has garnered ratings but has also left people fearing involvement with others. People worry that they might be taken advantage of or possibly put themselves in danger by stopping and helping someone who could really use some assistance.

Laziness impacts help simply because people don't often think about others' needs as much as their own desires. In 1961, U.S. President John F. Kennedy said in his inaugural address: "Ask not what your country can do for you; ask what you can do for your country."[2] These words spelled out the roots of a society, which is that everyone must pitch in to make this world prosper. Since that time, however, most politicians have repeatedly told citizens that government has failed the public, encouraging blame instead of participation. This has removed responsibility from people, causing them to believe that work should be done for them rather than by them. When these same people see someone in need, they don't even think to look past their own problems and help out their fellow human being. And everyone ends up suffering because of it.

Lastly, selfishness affects people's willingness to give to others because they believe it will take away precious time from themselves. Many modern innovations have increased the speed at which common tasks can be accomplished. While these advances have provided ways to get more done in less time, they have consequently influenced the desire to get more done in the day. By piling on more to do, it can seem like there aren't enough hours in the day to get everything done. And with this perception, many people refuse to give up what they feel they need more of: time.

When working on improving our own lives, sometimes we forget that others are doing the same. We get into a rhythm where we become focused on doing what we need to do and disregard anyone we believe is slowing us down from meeting our objectives. While recognizing patterns will give you good insight into the people who are habitually stalling your progress, every now and then, take a moment of your time to be patient with those you encounter. Check in with how they are doing and clarify your intentions. You can vastly improve your relationships by showing consideration for others rather than disregarding them simply because you have your own life to live. And who knows, you might even learn something.

The idea of help has been lost on so many of us. We don't seek help and avoid helping others. We shut ourselves off from the world. We focus on ourselves and mind our own business. But we're not alone in this world; it's just that we are surrounded by people who are similarly keeping to themselves. And until we start working together, we're all going to corner ourselves into depression.

The success of one is dependent on the help of many.

Chapter 16

Love:
The Gateway Emotion

Love is the language of poets. It is the subject of songs. People search for it. People die for it. It can overwhelm all rational thought. It nurtures the young and the old. It can be comforting and it too can be heart-wrenching.

I myself have felt my heart swell with emotion as I loved. I have given up my own plans for the love of another. I have turned my back on friends for someone else's love. I have been filled with rage toward those who sought to destroy my opportunity for mutual love. I have felt that I couldn't go on living without those I loved returning their love to me. I have refused to give up what I loved even when it was causing me continual pain.

And when I look back on the intensity of my love, I can barely tell the boundary distinguishing my love as an incredible display of affection or an incredible disregard of myself. It seems like those intense moments of love had my feelings teetering on an edge between seeing everything I wanted and losing everything I had.

But what is love really? Love is an emotion. It is the feeling of affection for another. It comes from inside you. However, love also feels like a connection, which causes most of us to think of love in terms of our relationships with others as a mutual feeling; but the emotions we feel are only our own. The strength of our love for others does not depend on whether those people love us in return. However, we typically interpret the quality of our love by the response it gets. We see the results of our love as confirmation of our own worthiness of love and validation that it's okay to love. And once again, we find our own emotions in the hands of other people by relying on their approval to tell us how to feel.

The truth is that all your emotions have a relationship to something. If you are scared of the dark, your relationship is with the dark. If you are angry with your friend, the relationship is between you and your friend. If you are proud of yourself, the relationship is with yourself. However, love is treated differently than other emotions because the meaning that people attribute to the love they feel causes them to attach so much of their being to it. As you recall, giving things too much meaning can lead to doubt, which is why so many people debate reasons why they should or shouldn't be in love, question whether to announce their love to another, or overanalyze whether someone is their perfect match. Unlike other emotions, love gets complicated by the significance attributed to it as people believe in concepts like finding "the one." But should love really be treated any differently than other emotions?

The answer is: Yes. Love *is* different because of the effect it has on other emotions. There are many levels of intensity with which we care. Sometimes we *like*; sometimes we *love*, and sometimes we're *in love*. And the intensity of our affection for someone or something is closely related to how easily our love leads us to feel other emotions, be them good or bad.

Some people call marijuana the gateway drug because they believe it leads to using other drugs. I consider love to be the gateway emotion because it leads to having other feelings. When you love, the other emotions you feel are linked positively or negatively to the way you feel about your love in that moment. And the more intense you feel about something, the more you'll be shaken by circumstances affecting it.

The Diagram of Love

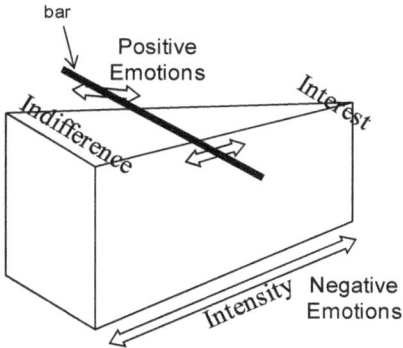

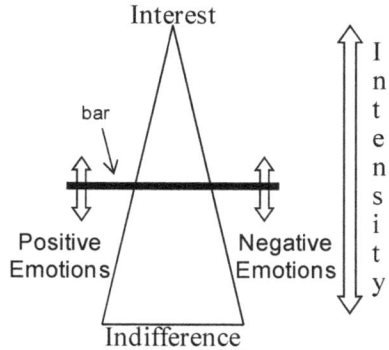

Consider these diagrams, which summarize my understanding of love. They are actually the same diagram, only shown from two different angles so you can more easily grasp the following concept. The wedge on the left is drawn three-dimensionally whereas the diagram on the right shows only the top side of the wedge on the left.

The wedge represents the object of your affection. The bar that lies on top of the wedge represents your feelings about what you love. This bar moves forward and back depending on how intense your feelings are. When you do not have much interest in someone or something, the bar lies near the widest part of the wedge (Indifference). As your feelings of love intensify, the bar moves up toward the point of the wedge (Interest).

Now you will also notice that on the left side of the wedge are written the words "Positive Emotions" and on the right side of the wedge are written the words "Negative Emotions." This is because the bar that lies on top of the wedge does not just move forward and back; it can also tip from side to side like a judicial scale. Logically, it makes sense that the closer the bar gets to the point of the wedge, where there is little support balancing the bar, the easier it becomes for the bar to tip to one side or the other. Depending on which side the bar is tipping toward, your general feelings and demeanor correspond with a positive or negative view of life. This is how your feelings about what you love lead to other emotions.

The more intense you feel about something or someone, the more volatile your emotions. For example, let's say you are very much in love with someone; and consequently the bar is near the point of "Interest" as shown in these diagrams:

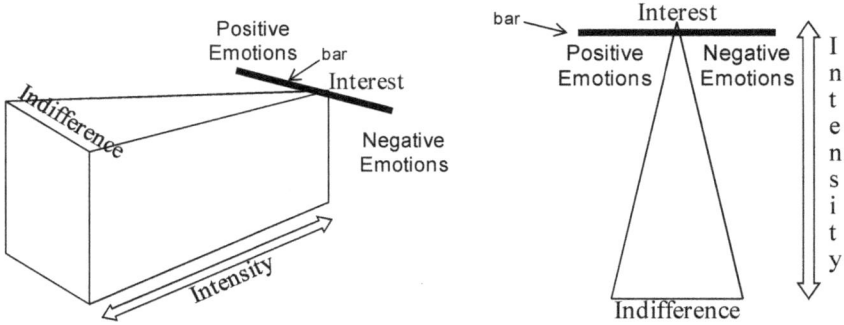

Because the bar is near the point of "Interest," there is less of a barrier between positive and negative emotions. Good and bad circumstances weigh down on the different sides of the bar and because of the lack of support to balance the bar level, the bar (your feelings) becomes easily susceptible to circumstances related to whom you care about.

So let's say that the person you love intensely did something that bothered you. With so little support balancing the bar, you would easily tip over to the "Negative Emotions" side, possibly feeling sad, angry, lonely, scared, and so on. Were that person to then do something nice for you, you might easily tip back over to the "Positive Emotions" side, feeling happy, confident, appreciative, or excited. This is not to say that certain emotions are good and others are bad. Rather, "positive" and "negative" emotions reference your own feelings of satisfaction or dissatisfaction with your life.

If the intensity of your love for that person was to drop and the bar moved toward the thicker part of the wedge, those same circumstances would be less likely to affect you. By not being as emotionally invested in that person, the bar rests over a much thicker area that provides it with more support, thereby giving your feelings more stability. So it would take a huge event with substantial weight to push your feelings to one side and feel particularly good or bad. And once that bar is tipped to one side, it would then take a lot to weigh down the other side of the bar to tip it over the huge section of the wedge to where the opposite emotions exist. However, you may not even notice these types of shifts in your feelings since your interest level is so low.

The song title "You Always Hurt the One You Love" has become a common expression for many people who have found truth in these words.[1] This is because as your love intensifies, your emotional state becomes less reliant on logic and more reliant on your circumstances. Have you ever gone from deeply loving someone when you are together to hating that person with all your being when you break up? Sometimes you don't even have to break up for those feelings to change. A simple argument can make you get uncharacteristically upset with someone you have strong feelings for.

This is primarily why people who love each other intensely often fight about insignificant issues. It takes so little to tip the bar from side to side when there is so little of the wedge stabilizing it. Because the bar tips quickly and easily, people often misinterpret those insignificant issues to hold a lot of weight. They don't; it's just the intensity of their love that makes their feelings sensitive to anything they are attached to. In love, you literally teeter between feeling good and feeling bad the more intense you feel about someone or something.

This diagram is not just about the love for another; it's about any type of love. This means that even self-love is represented by the diagram. The more significance, the more you doubt. The more intense, the more unstable. And this is why the people who are the most egotistical are so often the most insecure and often doubt everything they are doing. They tip from side to side, feeling good or bad based on what their circumstances suggest at the time about themselves because the intensity of their love affects the stability of their emotions.

Sometimes, because the edge is so thin near the point of the wedge, it is not only easy to tip from one side to the other; but you may not even know what side of the diagram you're on. For example, an intense love might make you feel as though you are willing to give up everything for the person you love. In a generous sense, this is a very caring action. From a reasonable point of view, however, this action shows a complete disregard for your own well-being. Because love is an emotion, the more intense it is, the less you use logic in making your decisions. So, in essence, the more intense your feelings are, the more the distinction between good and bad blurs.

The truth is that if I were to draw a Diagram of Hate, it would look nearly identical to the Diagram of Love. The only difference would be that instead of good circumstances related to the person you hate creating positive emotions within you, they would lead to negative emotions. Bad circumstances related to whom you hate would lead to positive emotions within you because of the inverse relationship between how you feel and how the person you hate feels.

The reason you hear phrases like "There's a thin line between love and hate" is not to suggest that if you hate someone, you borderline love that person. What the phrase points out is that the difference between the two is slight because both love and hate are emotional attachments. When you emotionally invest in someone or something, you put your emotions at risk in the interest of getting what you want in relation to your attachment. And the intensity with which you love or hate can have the same positive or negative impact on your feelings about the rest of you life.

Whether it is love or hate that you embrace, the problem is allowing an emotional attachment to take over your life. As you focus on what you are emotionally invested in, you bring more of what you are focusing on into your life. And eventually, if you continue to ignore reason and let emotion completely guide your focus, what you love or hate may not just feel like an attachment but an addiction.

How to Stabilize Your Love

In order to find the middle ground of healthy love, you need to learn how to balance your feelings. This requires answering the two big questions of what causes the bar to tip to one side or the other (to incite positive emotions in you or negative ones) and what moves the bar back and forth (in intensity).

We have already discussed what tips the bar from side to side: circumstances related to whatever you love. While you cannot control the world around you, it is not so much the circumstances alone that weigh down on your feelings though; it is your interpretation of those circumstances that gives them weight.

If a situation is presented that you determine to be bad, more weight is put on the negative side of the bar. If you interpret an experience as good, more weight is placed on the positive side of the bar. In addition to your personal interpretation of whether circumstances are good or bad, the more substantial you feel the circumstances are, the more weight they place on one side of the bar or the other.

Sometimes, however, your interpretation is not based on the severity of the circumstances themselves but on how intensely you feel about whom or what you love. As discussed already, when you love someone or something intensely and the bar is near the point, it doesn't take much to tip the bar. So you may interpret circumstances to be more substantial than they are because your intensity level allows inconsequential circumstances to tip the bar just as easily as circumstances that really matter.

This is where your other sense of control comes into play. When it comes to affecting the intensity of your love (moving the bar forward and back), your mind is what lowers it (moving the bar toward the wide end of the wedge) and your heart increases the intensity of your love (moving the bar closer to the point). Biologically, both emotion and reason originate in the brain; but for the purpose of explaining love, I will address the heart and the mind as separate controls by suggesting their connotative meaning of emotion and logic respectively. Your heart intensifies your feelings, but your mind, which is rational, serves the purpose of protecting you. Your mind understands intelligently that the higher you move up the wedge, the more volatile your emotional state will be; but your heart seeks the intensity of love. So following your heart intensifies the emotional experience of love while listening to your mind regulates it.

When it comes to balancing out their love, some people will try to control their love by using either their minds or their hearts to block out the other. They may use their minds to create a metaphorical wall around their hearts to stop themselves from feeling love for fear that they or someone else will get hurt. Or they might ignore the rationale of their minds to pursue what feels good in the moment. But in an effort to find balance, it's necessary not to jump to one extreme or the other. And to do that, you need to understand the reasons you love someone or something. Some people might tell you that some things just can't be put into words, but if you can't reasonably explain why you feel the way you do, you are definitely on the narrower part of the wedge. Knowing why you love another provides justification about your love to your mind while giving your heart permission to love.

You can't list all the reasons you love another because love is a feeling, not a thought. However, giving yourself reasons to love that correspond with your own values and desires gives both your heart and your head a place on the wedge where they can be in agreement. And only when your heart and your head are in agreement can your feelings about anything be both clear and at ease.

You have the ability to both feel and reason. One is not worse than the other. Both are abilities that you possess for the purpose of using them. Learning about yourself and the way you love is essential to creating stability and appreciation for what exists in your life.

True Love
Many people misunderstand what it really means to love. Often when people talk and think of love, it is selfish. It's "I"

this and "I" that. You might say, "I want to do this with you" or "I feel this way about you," but what about the other person? Love is not something you force upon another. Truly loving someone means honoring your feelings *and* allowing others to enjoy their own.

Consider the possibility that you love someone who doesn't love you back with the same intensity. Perhaps that person loves someone else. This might leave you feeling blue, trying to convince the person that a life with you would be wonderful.

This is not love, however. This is selfishness. Vying for someone else's love rather than allowing that person to do what he/she wants is just trying to convince that person to do what you want. Your desire for affection and to have someone accept your affection willingly does not always coincide with that person's desires. In true love, respect exists between those involved. If someone doesn't want to be with you, loving that person means respecting that choice. If you are unwilling to accept that person for who he/she is and what he/she wants and doesn't want, it probably means that you don't really love that person as much as you believe you do.

This understanding of love may help in dealing with problem relationships or love that isn't reciprocated because while your love may at times be selfish, you probably do care about the people you claim to love. I know it can still hurt when someone doesn't give you the type of affection you want in return for your affection, but if you truly love someone, encourage that person to do what he/she believes is right for him/herself.

Being Selfless Is Selfish

Every holiday season, it is said that "it is [better] to give than to receive."[2] This is because when you give to others, you are being thoughtful and you grow as a person. You learn the value of working toward making someone other than yourself feel good, and when you see the appreciation on another's face, you gain a good feeling in return. So, in a way, giving to others can sometimes double as a form of receiving. And this is similarly what people often do when they yearn for someone's love. They give and give, seeking to make someone else feel good because of their doing.

The problem is that, like with energy, it is equally important to give as it is to receive. If you try to always give to others because you care about those people while refusing to accept anything in return, you prohibit them from gaining the feelings and growth that come from giving. This can often lead to those people resenting you while you are left confused why anyone would despise you for being so caring. The fact is that just as giving can sometimes be a form of receiving, receiving from others is what allows those people to give of themselves and grow as individuals.

There is a story I once heard about a man who came upon a butterfly trying to emerge from its cocoon. He watched it for hours struggling to break free. So in an effort to help the butterfly, he used scissors to cut open the cocoon and set it free. What he did not realize, however, was that the struggle to emerge from the cocoon is what allows a butterfly to force its blood into its wings necessary for it to fly. The man inadvertently took away the butterfly's opportunity for growth through its own struggle and it never was able to fly.

People want to spend their time with others who make them feel good. Receiving is nice, but if someone takes away your opportunity for personal growth, that is not a person with whom you would want to spend your time. I've continued to stress the value of effort over results, and appreciation comes from effort, not from something that is just given. This is presumably why the term "Nice guys finish last" is so commonly used.[3] It isn't that being nice is bad; it's that giving so much that a person doesn't need to help him/herself creates a dependency that is commonly unappreciated.

Giving is not bad, but sometimes what you need to give people is the opportunity to grow. Help how you can without living others' lives for them. Let them give to themselves on occasion. You've got your own life to live.

Love and Depression

It is entirely possible to love others more than you love yourself, but what is important is that you love yourself *before* you begin expressing your love toward others. You may desperately want to share your life with someone right now, but if you are going through depression and don't appreciate yourself, now is not the time to be in a committed relationship. If you don't love yourself first, you can't have any idea how good your love is. And what kind of gift is your love for someone else if even you don't appreciate it?

People appreciate those who appreciate themselves. If you don't care about yourself, you are suggesting that there isn't any reason for others to care about you either. If you also give all your love to someone else, you put an unfair amount of pressure on that person to give you the love that you need in return.

Most people who are depressed haven't given up on love. They care about many people, just not the one who counts: themselves. They give all their love and energy away, making their happiness and self-esteem completely dependent on how others treat them. In a case like this, you don't love people because you care about them; you love them so that they will love you back in order to prove to you that you have value. You are consciously not caring about yourself but subconsciously seeking security. That's not love. That's selfishness.

Even if someone loves you, if you don't love yourself, that person will eventually give up on you. Your disregard for yourself will often outweigh the significance that you give to how others feel about you. So there becomes little anyone can say to please you. And those who love you will in time believe that their love is not enough and your love is too intense.

Now guess what happens when you don't love yourself and someone you've focused all your affection toward leaves you because you are constantly down about your life? You end up devastated because you feel like you have lost all the love that existed in your life. And you have lost all of it because you directed all the love you had away from you and are no longer getting any love returned to you. Loving yourself before loving another isn't just important for a relationship to thrive; it will be essential in helping you heal in case of a break-up.

What happens to some people is that they get into a relationship while feeling good about themselves, and the relationship goes well too. However, after receiving consistent admiration over time, they begin to rely on the other person in the relationship to validate them. Their self-love becomes dependent on another person, and a change in that person's affection for whatever reason leaves those people depressed. They then quickly seek love again from someone new, jumping from one relationship to another in order to regain self-esteem; but it rarely works. Sometimes they will chase the person that left them in an effort to regain confidence in themselves. But the fact is that until you love yourself, your happiness will always be dependent on how you believe others view you.

Unrequited Love

While love is an emotion that only you can feel, the idea of loving someone without that person loving you back can be crushing. This type of love is called unrequited love. The effects of unrequited love can be severely damaging to those who have not taken the time to love themselves first. Without self-love, when someone else does not return the love you give, unrequited love leads to devaluing your own self-worth. You are completely dependent on another person's affection to determine your own value, and you're not getting that affection. You dwell on how the other person doesn't want to be with you when you should be questioning why you want to be with that person. In all likelihood, if your love is unrequited, it is probably also infatuation. In these difficult times, it is often hard to see past your heart.

I remember a situation when I was in love with a girl who didn't want to be with me. She had gone camping with me and some friends, and I passed by her tent and noticed the shadow of a second figure inside. I just stood there staring at that tent, watching the shadows, forcing myself to accept the cold, hard truth that I had no chance with her. I realized while watching it how painful it was to me—how I was torturing myself willfully—but I couldn't look away, like when you can't stop staring at a terrible accident.

But there was another truth that I wasn't seeing. I wasn't seeing what existed everywhere else. In that tent, something was happening that I was interpreting. I was seeking some sort of confirmation that we couldn't be together that would allow me to move on, but I had an abundance of focus. I couldn't see all the great things in the world that were happening. I was only looking at one situation and accepting it as everything. Nothing else seemed to matter except what I was focusing on, but everything else does matter.

People feel unrequited love for what it is: a rejection of who they are. Unrequited love can be one of the most heartbreaking feelings, however, because it's not just a rejection of who you are; it is a rejection of who you are by someone you value. We seek loving relationships because of the good feelings that come from knowing someone loves and cares about us. So when someone you are fond of doesn't return the affection you offer, it can appear to be a suggestion that you are unworthy of love. In an effort to then feel important, you likely pine not so much for the person but for the person's approval. This can lead to putting up with abusive relationships, constant fighting, and giving up on your needs to make someone else happy.

Rejection can be difficult to bear, but refusing to accept rejection can cause you to fight for what you may not actually want. You may just want someone because you are told you can't have that person. What would happen if you got what you were fighting for, but it turned out that the only reason you wanted that person was because you were rejected? What if you just wanted confirmation that the person valued you, and once you got that, you realized you didn't really want a relationship with that person? You'd be stuck in a new uncomfortable situation. So before you fight for what you can't have, check in with yourself and be sure it's really what you want.

There is so much in this world worth appreciating. That one thing you can't have doesn't mean there is anything wrong with you, and it's not the only thing in your life. Take the time to look at your life objectively. You may want to suggest that nothing else matters besides what you want, but everything else you have does matter because that is where you will find those who approve of you.

Your self-esteem will play an important role in determining how hard you are hit by unrequited love. When you feel good about the person you are, you don't need confirmation of your merit. You may be disappointed when you don't get what you desire, but when you care about yourself, unrequited love doesn't overtake your focus. Your love for yourself is enough to prove that you have value.

Unrequited love is quite possibly the hardest personal challenge I faced in overcoming my own depression. I have also found that unrequited love plays a major role in most people's depression. Even some of the happiest people I know experienced their darkest days when pining for the love of someone else. Unrequited love involves having an abundance of focus, relying on hope, and refusing to accept reality. It involves so many ways of living that work against your growth and happiness.

In my own attempts to overcome the effects of unrequited love, I found the process to be a series of three techniques rather than just one. They involve 1.) Evaluating your relationship to the other person, 2.) Letting go of the other person, and 3.) Moving on by focusing on yourself.

Technique:
Extinguishing Unrequited Love (Part 1)

If you find yourself suffering from a bout of unrequited love, begin by turning to a blank page in your journal. Draw a vertical line down the center of the page, dividing it into two sections. On the left side, write down all the things that make you upset about the person you desire. Think hard. You will probably want to believe that the person is perfect, but try to think of disagreements and times you felt uncomfortable.

On the right side of the paper, write down all the things you want from a partner. Think hard about what is important to you. Don't think about characteristics the person you can't have possesses. Rather, concentrate on what you believe are valuable qualities that you would want in someone with whom you would commit to having a loving relationship. Then title the left column "What I'm Getting," and title the right column "What I Want."

What I'm Getting	**What I Want**
Typically running late	Wants to spend time with me
Complains often	Reliable
Broken many promises	Encouraging
Unwilling to compromise	Respects my point of view
Out of shape	Independent
	Accepting of my friends
	Wants to get married

Once you have written down your dissatisfactions with your love interest and what you want from someone in an intimate relationship, read over what you wrote. Recognize that the person you want may not be as perfect as you felt a moment earlier. Also, take note of how that person may not possess many of the qualities you desire in a lover. Just to start, I'll give you one area of disconnect. One of the characteristics that would likely be important in someone you want to be with would be that the person wants to share his/her time with you. If that person doesn't want to be with you, then he/she is probably not giving you what you want. The people you love should make you happy, and unrequited love does not invoke happiness.

Your list does not have to be nice; it only needs to be truthful. If physical appearance is important to you and the person you have unrequited love for is not that attractive, write this quality down on your list and compare it to what you want in a partner. Like everything in your journal, this list is personal; and you should be honest. You need to separate the person from your pattern emotions to determine if that person's qualities represent what you really want.

Keep in mind that no one will ever be perfect and fulfill all your desires. You will have to let go of less important requirements and accept that people make mistakes. However, when it comes to wanting what you can't have, take the time to determine what matters to you rather than what is merely in your view.

———

The purpose of this technique is to bring your head back into the equation so that you can recognize what you simultaneously feel and think about a person. When you suffer from unrequited love, your rational thoughts are typically overwhelmed by your emotional attachment, barring you from seeing how certain people might not be good fits for you. You may tend to disregard anything negative about someone, focusing only on that person's good qualities. You need to come back to reality because although that is a nice way to treat someone, by denying that anything negative about the person matters to you, you are not treating yourself well.

It's important to understand why you crave someone so badly, and this technique may show you that it has little to do with what the person you desire can provide you. If there are only a few similarities between what you want in a partner and what the person you love would provide, consider other possibilities for your infatuation. Is the reason for your attachment familiarity? Is it not wanting to feel rejected and, therefore, wanting what you can't have? Does the person represent something or someone else? Ask yourself questions so that you can understand the role that *you* play in your love, not just the role that the person you love plays.

Just because you may realize that what you want for your life and what someone can provide you are different, this does not bar you from caring about that person. It does, however, require that you face the reality of the situation. It's okay to love people, but it's not always best for you to maintain close relationships with them. Accepting both your feelings for someone else and your compatibility with that person is not always easy when the two contradict each other, but it's essential that you know there is nothing wrong with how you feel. And knowing that it's okay to feel the way you do makes the effort required in separating yourself from someone you love much easier.

The realization that someone isn't right for you may come after someone rejects you, or this realization may cause you to give up someone whom you are still in a relationship with. In either case, you realize what is right for you when you examine what you are getting and what you want. You look at the circumstances and the people involved because, as you recall, those are the two ingredients that make a relationship work.

Part of the draw of unrequited love and the continuation of infatuation is the thought that the person you seek may come around after a while and exhibit all the characteristics you want, including the desire to be with you. It is possible that this could happen, but all you have is now. Whether or not the person changes in the future is irrelevant. At the time when you are faced with a dilemma, you have to make a decision as to whether you are willing to wait around for a future that may never come or determine that what you are searching for must be addressed now.

Think about those in whom you invest your energy. Do they make you feel good about yourself? Do they make you work to be a better person? Sometimes people have served a particular purpose in your life, and now it's time to move on to new experiences with those people or without them.

Technique:
 Shifting Your Emotional Perspective (Part 2)

Part 2 of *Extinguishing Unrequited Love* is taking the understandings that you gained from the previous technique and applying those lessons to your life. Anything you learn in this world is only as valuable as your commitment to incorporating it into how you live. So let's take your realizations a step further by applying them to your life.

This process begins by thinking about what *the person you love* wants. Just like how with true love, you care about what the other person wants, you need to display that consideration now. The way to show consideration for another's feelings is to accept them. And when you accept what is causing a situation, you consequently accept the situation as well.

Take a moment and think about what the person whose affection you long for wants to do with his/her own life. Maybe the person wants to move away, spend time with someone you don't like, or simply not spend time with you. Whatever it is that the person wants to do with his/her life, simply take a moment to think about it.

Once you have considered the interests of this person, begin saying out loud how you are okay with him/her pursuing those interests and what it means for your own life. Start saying phrases like, "I am okay with this person pursuing what he/she wants," "I am okay with this person being happy," "I am okay without this person in my life," or "I am okay with continuing to search for love."

Once you admit your acceptance of whatever the person wants and may already be doing, then explain to yourself why you are okay with it. You've got a whole list of reasons from Part 1. Remember, you are bringing your mind back into the picture; and your mind works on logic. Once you tell yourself the reason, again come back to telling yourself out loud, "I am okay with..."

The idea here is accepting that because of the reasons you wrote down in Part 1, you are okay with another person leading his/her life however he/she chooses. You are not lying to yourself. You are simply convincing yourself to believe what you already know to be true. You are breaking through to yourself. You are not convincing yourself to be someone you're not; you are embracing a part of yourself that you forgot about.

This technique is not meant to be disingenuous. Too many people believe that the heart is genuine and that the mind plays tricks on you. The truth is that what you think and how you feel are both important parts of who you are and one shouldn't be used to silence the other. Rather, they should help each other so that they are on the same page. You must think and feel the same way to be at peace.

It's important to know what someone does or doesn't provide you, and it's important to know what you want. And just as you want to have and do what you want, others need that opportunity also. Letting others do what they want to do without making a fuss is all part of accepting this world. Still, there is something that is missing from the equation of unrequited love; it's who you are irrespective of the person you desire.

Technique:
Who You Are without Another (Part 3)

In Part 2 of this three-part technique in overcoming the effects of unrequited love, you began admitting that you are okay with someone living his/her life as he/she pleases. You took the time out of your own life to think about and accept what another person wants to do with his/her own life. Now it's time to give yourself that same respect.

Just as you considered what the person you desire wants to do, think about what *you* want to do. But here's the catch: you have to think about something you want to do that doesn't involve the person you love. You don't have to decide what you want to do for the rest of your life. That's not the purpose of this technique. You just have to think about something you want to do completely unrelated to that person. Maybe you want to travel, go to school, pick up a new hobby, or write a book.

Once you have thought of at least one thing that you want to do with your life irrespective of the person you love, realize that just as that person wants to do what he/she wants to do, you should do what you want to do. This is an opportunity to do something you might not have otherwise done. By focusing on a new objective, you help yourself to refocus your energy away from something you can't have to something you can have. The person holding you back from moving on with your life is not someone who doesn't want you; with unrequited love, you're the one stopping yourself from moving on.

You've taken the opportunity to write down what you want to fill the spot of a lover in your life. Now it's time to pursue what you want out of the other areas of your life. When you are infatuated, you see so much of your life related to whom you love; but by taking on a new activity unrelated to your infatuation, what you do makes you someone independent from the person you love. It makes you an individual in charge of creating your own life. You are not your relationships. Relationships are just something you have, and when it comes to your relationship with yourself, it's up to you to determine what you are going to do with what you have.

———

When your feelings overtake your mind, you lose a part of yourself. As humorous as it may sound, in the case of unrequited love, you've lost your mind. When you think about it though, the lack of logic that exists in the actions of someone intensely in love is very similar to descriptions of insanity. In fact, we often describe intense love in language that references insanity. "I am crazy about you," "He raves about her," "She is mad about him," "You drive me out of my mind," or "I am wild about you" are all common ways of describing one's intense love for another.

When you've lost the role of your mind in the equation of love, you need to regain all of who you are. Look inward, accept the moment, and realize that you are more than just a companion; you are an individual with great possibility. Once you refocus on this fact, what you want just might change; and a change in desire is a change in emotion. And that's how you take charge of your life after infatuation turns ugly.

Love can feel wonderful, and sometimes it can feel agonizing. Love leads to a variety of emotions that become increasingly vulnerable to your surroundings as the intensity of your love grows. And while vulnerability might give you opportunities in which you learn to trust people, in a world in which change is a constant, you don't want to live every moment of your life that way.

When you allow yourself to feel love openly yet take the time to understand why you feel the way you do, you bring balance to your love. Without that balance, you end up emotionally unstable, ignoring how you feel in your heart or disregarding what you know in your mind is best for you. Both your heart and your mind are key players in love, and using one to hide the other is not being genuine. It's only when you use all of who you are to express your love that you give your love value.

The way you love affects all your emotions. So when it comes to your happiness, loving yourself comes first. It's your first and last relationship, and it's one you're constantly affected by. Only once you love yourself will your love for another be an extension of your character, not a representation of it. And so equally important as how you love others is how you love yourself: by using both your head and your heart, knowing exactly why you care about the person that you are.

Don't let your love be how you express your fear of rejection.

Chapter 17

Managing Your Relationships

You have relationships with everyone and everything you encounter. It's just that some of those relationships are going better than others. Depression is a consequence of a bad relationship with yourself, but because we often approach different aspects of our lives in the same way, a bad relationship with yourself means you probably have bad relationships with a lot of people. Those people may not always see it that way, but you probably feel like they do.

So what is it that you must have to maintain healthy relationships in your life? What is it that you have lost in the relationship with yourself? What is it that must be the cornerstone of every relationship? The answer to all these questions is the very important element of a relationship called "Respect."

Every type of relationship at its core must have respect to flourish. Whether it is friendship, romantic love, a job, or even driving a car, it all comes down to respect for yourself and for whom or what you have the relationship with. Love, trust, and appreciation all breed from respect. So too do attentiveness, etiquette, and commitment grow out of respect. In order for an animal to trust you, you must show it respect. In order not to get burned when lighting a match, you must respect the fire. The same is true with humans. It is up to you to have and show respect for others in order to receive the same from them. Wanting respect before giving it is backward.

So what does it mean to respect someone else? It means taking into consideration that person's feelings and accepting that person as he/she is. When you respect someone, you show an interest in that person's well-being. You realize that the person may have perspectives that differ from yours without viewing that person's feelings as less important than your own.

When the respect is mutual, the other person values your perspectives as well. And when two varying perspectives are respected by two different people, these people can grow together as it is respect that makes the exchange of energy that exists in all strong relationships possible and valuable.

Exploring Your Relationships

Part of the methodology within this guide has been to help you appreciate everything with value in your life while eliminating everything that distracts you from that. However, before you can really appreciate what you have, you must know what you have. Titles exist in most relationships, but titles also mean different things to different people. So if you don't explore and learn about the relationships you have, you might get caught off guard in ways you never expected. Someone might unintentionally treat you differently than how you believe your title suggests you should be treated. And the same goes for how you treat others.

If you believe that the titles that exist between you and another person mean that you should be treated or act in a specific way, discuss your feelings with that person. Just like with the "Checking In on Change" technique, see how that person views the relationship. Ask what he/she wants to get out of the relationship with you. Find out where he/she foresees the relationship headed. This way, you prevent yourself from misinterpreting the type of relationship you have, and you may even open up the possibility of taking your relationship to a new level.

When you explore your relationships, you are not focusing on what might happen but what is happening now. This means that rather than telling someone how to act, you discuss each other's feelings and comfort levels. For example, rather than demanding that someone you are dating be faithful to you or simply expecting that the person believes in monogamy, find out how that person interprets the boundaries and openness of your relationship with each other.

Remember that when someone explains his/her beliefs, feelings, or desires, LISTEN! So many people are told answers they don't want to hear, and so they just ignore them as if those words didn't matter. When someone talks to you, listen and take what you are told to heart. Otherwise, you'll pursue what doesn't exist while failing to acknowledge what does. And a relationship like that has an impending expiration date.

One of the greatest parts about a relationship is getting to know the person. Take the time to learn about where you are investing your energy. It's the exploration and understanding of beliefs, feelings, and desires that will prepare you for the future much better than demanding, hoping, and expecting. Only once you know what you have, can you know whether it's something you truly appreciate.

As you explore your relationships with others, you will expose yourself to the reality of possibilities. Exploration will open doors for some relationships as you discover that both you and another person want to develop your relationship to a deeper level. However, exploration will also close doors for some relationships as you encounter conflicting interests in the present or future intensity of a relationship. What you want in a relationship may not be what another person wants. And the highest level of commitment that can exist in a relationship at any one point is the same as the lowest level of commitment that either person is willing to make. For example, if you want to date someone but that person only wants to be friends, the most you can be is friends. No relationship can ever be more than it is unless both people want to explore the boundaries of that bond. But you will never know what's possible unless you learn how the people with whom you have relationships feel.

Whether a door is opened or closed by looking into your relationships, you get the opportunity to learn about what you have in your life: the depth, the limits, and the possibilities. You learn about the shared views and disconnect on what each of you value. In any lasting relationship, you don't have to agree on everything (and you won't); but what matters is that you agree on what is most important to each of you. Personal desires may change over time, but if what you and your partner most want to do with your lives imposes on each other's plans, resentment may develop and the relationship will eventually deteriorate.

Filling the Voids

Each of us has a great deal we can contribute to this world, but none of us are complete. We all have missing pieces from our lives, often represented by areas in which we need improvement, assistance, or nurturing. These pieces may be missing from your own life from having given of yourself without getting anything in return, never having had particular experiences, or change taking place. Regardless of the reasons behind such missing pieces, relationships are one of the primary ways to fill these voids in your life and create a feeling of completion.

There is more to relationships than simply getting along with people and tolerating their lesser points while they tolerate yours. A relationship is an exchange of goods, services, or feelings. It is an interaction and an exchange of energy. The relationships that last are the ones that continually distribute what everyone in the relationship needs; in other words, those relationships have the right people and the right circumstances.

A teacher might offer you knowledge; a job might offer money, or a friend might offer a helping hand. And the relationships that offer the things you need are likely to be the ones you value and keep. While many relationships will provide you with benefits, it's important to know that no single relationship will ever provide all the missing pieces in your life. Different people have different purposes in your life. Even a spouse cannot be everything to another person. If you rely on another to fill all the voids in your life, the relationship will disintegrate prematurely.

When you think about it though, would you really want one person to fill all the voids in your life? It's risky to your own well-being. It creates an abundance of focus in your life. Again, you are faced with the concept of putting all your eggs in one basket if your best friend, your lover, and your business partner, for example, are the same person. You lose the person and you lose them all. You'll immediately feel the emptiness of all those voids and almost instantaneously fall into depression.

No one person will ever give you everything you want. Other relationships, including the one you have with yourself, are there to fill in the gaps. Every relationship in your past and present life has helped to shape the person you are today. Relationships of all levels—from friends to love interests, relatives and even enemies—play different roles in your life. And it's important not to confuse these roles. You cannot treat your spouse like you treat your parents and you cannot treat your child like you treat your pet. Everyone in your life is playing a role.

Not everyone will fit into the roles you want, however. Someone may not make a good lover but is an excellent friend. Someone may be an excellent friend but a terrible roommate. You will experiment with different types of relationships with different people throughout your life, and some will work while others will fail because of whether they possess the right people and the right circumstances for that type of relationship.

Similarly, you cannot fill all the voids in the lives of those with whom you have relationships. You do, however, serve important purposes in their lives. But if you're not playing a specific role in someone's life, it is possible that the person will seek out from someone else what he/she is not getting from you. This means nothing against you. It simply means that people will seek out those missing pieces in their lives however they can. If you don't have any interest in playing a specific role in someone's life, it shouldn't matter that the person chose another to help him/her out. However, many people get upset because of jealousy.

You don't have the energy or the time to participate in everything, filling everyone's voids while trying to pay attention to your own. Instead, it's best that you give your time and energy to what you feel are the most important and enjoyable aspects of your relationships for yourself and for others.

Growth in Relationships

Even if a relationship fills in some missing part of your life, what matters is not what you get but what you do with what you get. And your opportunity in a relationship is to acquire the tools someone provides you to improve your own life regardless of whether the relationship lasts.

Those in your life who are filling your voids are also offering you opportunity. They are offering you the opportunity to take what they are giving you and grow because of it. Just as many of the relationships you once had in your life no longer exist, what someone else offers you now will probably not always be around. And if you don't take advantage of the opportunity to learn and grow, you may continue to seek the same things from different relationships.

Let's say, for example, that you don't have any love for yourself; and so you disregard what you truly want in a partner just to fill the void of love in your life. In a case like this, you are using the relationship to provide the missing piece of love within your life; but the relationship may not be helping you grow. If you're not taking the love someone offers you and equally learning to appreciate yourself, the relationship is merely compensating. Were it to end, you would still be missing love for yourself and would, therefore, continue to seek out nothing more than love from someone new without any regard for the other voids in your life.

In any relationship, it's important to know what you are giving, know what you are getting, and grow because of the help of another. That way, you no longer need someone else to fill the same voids in your life repeatedly. Instead, you learn to rely on yourself, rounding out those missing pieces in your life so that you can take the next step of focusing on other areas of your life that need work. We have so much to share and so much to gain, and using your relationships as opportunities for growth helps relationships continue because you and your companions end up growing together.

People often want to be in control of their relationships. They want to be the popular ones, determining the course of their relationships; but this leadership role comes with a considerable loss to their ability to grow. If you believe that you are better at most things than those around you, it's time to change who you are hanging out with because you aren't going to learn much. You will give to others while not appreciating what they provide you. And when the relationships dissolve because of your voids not being filled, you might feel like you wasted your life because you gave of yourself without getting anything of value in return.

While you certainly have a great deal of knowledge within you, you can also learn a lot from those around you who can teach you what they know. If a relationship exists between you and another person, take the time to learn from that person. That way, even if the relationship goes sour or the person leaves, you will have gained something that you can take with you for the rest of your life. Have you ever seen those shirts that say, "I did _____ and all I got was this lousy t-shirt"? Well, you should be getting something from your relationships that you can take with you, be it knowledge, talent, skills, a new friend, or valuable experiences. That's the whole point of creating a connection: to improve your life.

Take pleasure in not always being right. It gives you the opportunity to learn about yourself and this world in which you live. Take pleasure in that not being the center of attention means you have a better opportunity to gain new skills, realizations, and experiences than you would have had if you were "number one." If you have everything, you have nothing to gain.

Conflict

Any relationship will have complications at times, and when disagreements arise, people sometimes reevaluate their relationships. Many people want the perfect relationship in which they never fight, but demanding perfection is a symptom of extremism and, as discussed, will lead right to depression. Seeking the perfect relationship will cause you agitation at the first sign of discontent. So it will ease your frustration to know that conflict is both inevitable in relationships and serves a very important role in personal growth.

First, let's explore conflict. All conflicts are based on judgment. Think of any disagreement you've ever had in your life. It was based on your judgment of what was appropriate conflicting with someone else's point of view.

Now think about those people with whom you have the most conflict. They are likely the people who affect your life the most. Even if those people are whom you care about, you judge them more than others because you believe their behavior could most significantly impact your livelihood in positive or negative ways.

While conflict may seem like a negative consequence of relationships, it is a key way that you learn and grow. Conflict exposes you to different perspectives that provide the opportunity to enhance your knowledge about yourself and this world. And when open to new perspectives, you have new experiences that can open up doors for you regardless of whether you stay in a relationship for the long term. You gain knowledge about life that no one can ever take away from you.

You don't need to agree with everything you are presented, but conflict only feels abrasive because it conflicts with what you believe to be correct. Any struggle against another's perspective is just your fear of losing your comfort zone for a new way of life. However, there are many ways of living your life and many ways to view this world. Other people can open your eyes to those possibilities.

If you agreed with someone all the time or someone always agreed with you, the relationship would eventually grow stale. If you truly care about someone and believe that person has something to share, consider the person's point of view and question your own. Respecting others and yourself means being open to considering both what you believe and what someone else believes.

Conflicts present opportunities to view the world in new ways and to better get to know someone with whom you are investing your life. By understanding new perspectives, you both learn. You grow together rather than forcing each other to conform. And truthfully, if you are not gaining new knowledge from your relationships or having your perspectives considered, there may be an absence of self-respect or an absence of mutual respect for each other's beliefs.

Of course, the big issue with conflict that makes it valuable or destructive is how it is resolved. Is it used as an opportunity for growth by addressing underlying themes in your relationship or does the conflict end simply because both people are tired of arguing? Does one person give in or do both people come away with new perspectives? A positive resolution of conflict comes down to being open to questioning your own beliefs, respecting each other's opinions, and accepting change within the relationship.

Having a relationship with anyone else will require you to make some sacrifice. It means you will have to consider others in your decision making. This may at times feel like a burden, but learning to interact with those around you is all part of learning to make the most of your life in a world in which you are not alone.

This is where the concept of compromise comes into play. Now I used to hate compromising. I saw it as me giving up my independence, desires, and freedom. However, in order to compromise without feeling bad, you must explore a situation and yourself to determine what aspect of an issue is most important to you. And that is what you must maintain as part of a compromise. Everything else is secondary. In order to compromise effectively, focus strictly on what matters to you rather than circumstantial details so that both people can grow from the conflict.

While conflict is an inevitability that can provide great insight into your relationships and yourself, it's important to determine when conflict stops providing opportunities for growth and starts making your life more difficult to grow. When you encounter the same problems with people repeatedly, conflict is not serving a constructive purpose. Typically in these situations, you are only able to see two visions: the situation as you want it to be and the situation as it is now. However, repeating negative events are simply part of patterns; and you have to change your behavior to change a pattern. The following technique alleviates the confusion of how to deal with persistent problems in life by laying out your only real options.

Technique: Solving Ongoing Problems (The 4-Option Technique)

You have four options for addressing any <u>ongoing</u>, difficult situation in your life.

Options:
A. Accept the situation as it is.
B. Do something about the situation to alleviate what is bothering you.
C. Request that someone change the situation.
D. Leave your surroundings.

To begin this technique, first ask yourself if the situation involves material things or is something that really isn't that big of a deal in the grand scheme of life; essentially, can you live sanely with the situation as it stands? Your immediate answer will likely be "No," but take a moment to really consider the significance of the situation. If you realize you can live with it or are willing to learn to live with it, you have your answer. It is Option A: you accept the situation as it is and get on with your life. If not, move on to Option B.

If you are unable to let a situation continue as it is without feeling agitated, your second option is to work toward improving your circumstances. This may mean finding a way to circumvent the issue that is bothering you or fixing the situation yourself. So much of life is the effort you put forth, and in many ongoing conflicts, the best action may be to just do something about the situation yourself, resolving the issue quickly in the best way you can. However, if you believe that the problem is too big for you to fix, it is out of your hands, or you have handled similar situations too many times in the past to be content fixing the problem yourself, move on to Option C.

If you moved on to Option C, politely ask someone to handle the situation. There are several ways to accomplish this, but any method must involve being both respectful and direct. A few good ways to ask for favors are to start off your request with: "I would appreciate it if you would…" or "I'd really prefer it if you would…" In each of these examples, you begin a statement in which you request a favor without asking a question and, therefore, do not offer the person the opportunity to respond with a simple "yes" or "no." Furthermore, you are not so much demanding someone change as you are expressing how you would feel if the person fixed the problem.

A second approach is to simply explain how the person's current actions make you feel and why you feel the way you do. This is also often effective because you are again focusing on how the situation affects you rather than demanding someone else change. You are counting on the person's respect for your feelings to influence him/her to change.

Yet another approach that is frequently met with successful results is to compliment someone before explaining your feelings about an issue that might be met with defensiveness. For example, you might say, "I love you, but I think it's about time that you…" or "I think you're a great person, but it would mean a lot if you would…"

You can even try compromising or working together with the person to alleviate the negativity of the situation. And this experience might allow you to feel better both about the situation and the relationship.

All of these methods open up the lines of communication and use respect to encourage some or all of the work be done by another. You don't have to use any of the methods I have suggested, but remember that the point of encouraging a favor is to have someone help out. So avoid sarcasm or negativity in the tone of your voice when making the request or it will change the connotation of the approach entirely.

While situations may not always be handled to your liking, it's important to determine if the effort that someone makes is enough to let go of the negativity the situation is creating for you. You may find it necessary to explain to the person that not getting what you want will cause you to walk away from the relationship, but only do this if you truly feel that way. By making it clear that the relationship is at risk and why, you open up a final chance for resolution before an exit. Your value to that person may encourage him/her to give you what you need to make the relationship worthwhile to you. Give the person a chance, and take notice of what is done. If the person honors your request, problem solved. If not, reconsider Option B (handling the situation yourself).

The reason to reconsider Option B is because Option D ends an experience, removing not just the bad but also the good. The objective of this technique is finding a way to move forward with your life. While leaving behind the good to get rid of the bad may be the right decision, it's important to learn how to work with people rather than impulsively giving up and walking away from them.

However, when you have attempted the first three options without success and you have reached your breaking point, you must move on to Option D and leave. Option D is not simply ignoring a situation but allowing it to affect your life so much that you feel the only solution is to walk away. Walking away may mean giving up an experience, ending a relationship, or possibly leaving town. You determine the extent to which you must leave your surroundings in order to move on with your life. The level of drama involved in walking away will be directly related to the emotional attachment of those involved in the situation. The less intense those in the relationship feel about the relationship and its circumstances, the easier Option D will be on those involved.

Leaving your surroundings may at times make you feel as though things resolved unfairly. This is why Option D is a last resort, but it is still an option. It may be exactly what is needed to move on and leave the past behind you, but it is also helpful to know what you are walking away from.

—

Calling It Quits

If your use of "The 4-Option" technique led you to Option D and the decision to walk away from a relationship, the following scale will give you one final chance to evaluate if it is truly the best decision for you. Evaluation is all part of exploring your options, and it can play a significant role in preventing you from second-guessing yourself.

Relationship Scale of Finality

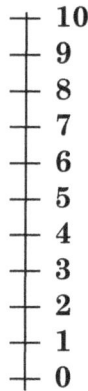

10
9
8
7
6
5
4
3
2
1
0

Because leaving a relationship with anyone or anything of importance can be a major decision, it will benefit you to first consider whether it is better or worse to give up what you have to avoid the stress caused by unresolved issues within a relationship. The first step in making your decision is determining the value of the relationship. The Relationship Scale of Finality ranges from 0-10 in order for you to rate your relationship. 10 represents getting everything you want from the relationship and 0 represents not getting anything at all. Rarely in life does anything rate a 10 or 0. In all likelihood, if you think that a relationship has a value of 10 or 0, you are looking at the relationship from a bad perspective. 10's are usually based on addictions or infatuations, and 0's are typically the result of sadness or anger over a recent incident.

Concentrate on how the good and the bad make you feel. Everyone and everything has good and bad points, and to be able to make good decisions about the direction of your life, you need to be able to see both of them. Once you've rated the value of your relationship, consider if that value is better or worse than having nothing.

As an example, say you don't like your job. You don't like going and you don't feel appreciated. If you have tried accepting the situation as it is (Option A), working hard (Option B), and speaking to your boss (Option C), then rate the relationship on the scale. Let's say you give it a 3. That's pretty low, but it's not as low as 0. Even though you may want your job to be a 10, you are reasonable and would probably be willing to settle for a 7. The problem is that 7 isn't a choice; it doesn't exist.

Because you already attempted three of the four options to change your circumstances before considering the scale, you are left with just two places on the scale that your job's value can be: 3 or 0. You can remain at the job as things are, with both the good that made its rating a 3 and the bad that kept it from being any higher. Or you can walk away, leaving your relationship nonexistent with a consequential rating of 0. This is your only decision. If you are unhappy, leave the relationship; but decide for yourself first if nothing is better or worse than how things presently stand. Leaving an experience will give you more time and energy to concentrate on other things, but it also removes all the good features that come with the experience. Which is more important to you?

Whatever you decide, be true to yourself. Never stay in a situation because you are afraid of living without it. Good experiences will come in time. Leaving any relationship that consistently makes you unsatisfied may be the right decision for you to take charge of your life. If I hadn't done it, you wouldn't be reading this book.

Many times people will choose to walk away from situations, but when they give up what they have, only then does it seem like the little they had was a lot. And it was a lot compared to the nothing that they took instead. Even if a relationship in your life rates a 1 on the scale, the relinquishment of the relationship means the loss of an attachment. While this may be good in the long run, you may feel a sense of loss and fear of how to fill the new void in your life. Even change that comes from within you can be scary because it is a step in a new direction. That fear is over the uncertainty of the future.

It's important to remember in times of second-guessing that there were reasons that guided your decision. A decision like leaving a relationship is intense enough that you very likely addressed it in your journal. Turn to your own writing when you question your past decisions to remind yourself why you made them.

In the end, you always walk away from relationships. All this means is that at some point, you stop feeling an attachment to the relationship, even if that point comes when you die. Sometimes you have the feeling of disconnecting before others; sometimes you move on long after they walk away, and sometimes the decision is mutually agreed upon. But your feelings change when you are ready, never before and never after despite what you might prefer.

Every relationship's success comes down to the right people and the right circumstances, and often it is people's respect for each other's circumstances that makes them both "right." Respect is what allows for exploration into your life and your relationships as well as understanding of what you discover in that exploration. Respect is what allows conflict to be a tool for growth. It is what allows you to make good decisions for yourself by accepting and appreciating what exists in this world.

There are many types of relationships that will come in and go out of your life, and every relationship will provide different opportunities for you. Sometimes they will be opportunities that you were seeking. Other times, they may be opportunities to prove your capabilities to yourself as you strive to overcome unanticipated challenges. Regardless, the voids in your life only remain filled beyond the moment of the experience if you are able to take what you gain from one relationship with another into your relationship with yourself.

The more people argue over who is right and who is wrong, the further they distance themselves from any opportunity for peace.

Chapter 18

Communication

There are two common problems that many people, particularly those unsatisfied with their lives, have when it comes to their interactions with others. These problems are blowing things out of proportion and the inability to communicate effectively. Let's tackle blowing things out of proportion first.

Not everything is that big of a deal and worth stressing over. Whether it is someone who was rude to you, a friend who didn't call you back, or a bad restaurant waiter, most things that get people irritated aren't life or death. In fact, next time something upsets you, consider how likely the situation is to be on your mind when you are lying on your deathbed.

The reason we get upset over certain situations is because of the way we interpret them. Interpretation is subjective. For example, rain to a farmer might be good; but rain to a bride on her wedding day might be bad. Does that mean that one of these viewpoints is wrong? No. What it means is that *we* give things meaning. The farmer or bride may love or hate the rain, but it doesn't change the fact that it's just rain. Moreover, their opinions don't change whether it rains; their opinions only change the way they feel. How you interpret your circumstances is how an experience affects you.

When it comes to the things in life that upset you, it's important to understand why they bother you. I encourage you to use the "Questions" technique from Chapter 6 to get down to the root of your beliefs and feelings about whatever upsets you. Once you understand and accept what about a situation actually bothers you, you can take control of it by addressing only the parts of the situation that really matter.

There are many paths in life to get to what matters to you. When you take the time to consider the reasons behind why you want things to be a particular way, you can then focus on other ways to address those reasons in your life. Your responsibility to yourself is to recognize the difference between what matters and what is just a path to what matters.

Let's start by determining what matters.

Technique: Setting Your Priorities

Turn to a blank page in your journal. Write down on this page the most important things you can think of in your life. Be specific. Include your goals, interests, friends, or whatever you greatly value. When you are done, title the top of the page, "My Priorities."

Now read over your list. I'll wait.

——

What is on your list is what is worthy of your attention. I'm guessing you didn't write something down like keeping track of your keys. If this is the case, the next time you get upset about misplacing your keys, remember that you didn't put that on your list as something important to you.

When you encounter frustrating situations, however, you may try to create associations between unimportant circumstances and your priorities. For example, you might believe that losing your keys would make you late for work, which could cause you to lose your job that you need for money; and money gives you freedom, which is a priority of yours. The relationship between losing your keys and having freedom is simply cause and effect, but you can connect any event to another if you try hard enough. Your problems, however, are not always closely tied to your priorities. Rather, it is typically you creating the link.

Let's take a closer look at the associations you create in your life that cause you frustration by taking the previous example. By breaking down the connection between the visible problem and your priority, we see the following parts:

Lost Keys → Transportation to Job → Job Security → Money → Freedom

What breaking down this connection does is show how indirect the relationship is between your keys (the issue upsetting you) and your freedom (your priority). What is more important though is recognizing that even if you lost your keys, your freedom may have not yet been compromised. So nothing exceptionally bad may have even taken place.

But breaking down the association into its separate parts has a bigger purpose than just displaying how indirect the relationship is between the visible problem and your priority. It also shows you the different ways in which you can take charge of the situation in order to address your priority before anything bad actually happens. While finding your keys may be out of your control, you could find different transportation to work, call your job and let them know you are running late, choose to spend or save your money differently, or take some time to consider what freedom really means to you. While it is easy to blame the most visible reason for why you feel frustrated, there are often many ways to attend to your priorities.

The control you have over your priorities is often much greater than you realize or utilize. People often create elaborate associations between circumstances out of their control and priorities in their control. Getting upset about misplacing your keys neither helps you find your keys nor puts your attention on the bigger picture of what really matters. Your control is in how you handle situations, and once you address one aspect of the association to affect your priority, the inconvenience at hand no longer seems that big of a deal.

These types of associations are common for many people who exhibit a pattern of blowing things out of proportion. They fail to see how much control they have over their happiness, instead focusing on even the smallest problems as hurdles in their way of being happy. They are constantly fighting, and it is precisely that fight inhibiting their happiness.

Many people get upset over trivial obstacles because in some way, they feel it is their duty to not just maneuver around them but to fix them. However, your list of priorities acknowledges what is important in your life while everything else isn't worth nearly as much of your attention. Ask yourself questions about your priorities so that you understand why they are important to you. Your priorities will change throughout your life. So update your list often. Give yourself the opportunity to relax by being aware of what truly matters to you and what is truly no big deal.

Passive-Aggression: How It Works and Why It Fails

The second common problem that people typically have in their interactions with others is their inability to communicate effectively. Rarely is it what people say that affects others; it is more often the approach they use. The manner in which you choose to communicate with others will determine just how effective you are in communicating your thoughts and feelings. Misunderstandings, defensiveness, and indifference can often be the result of ineffective methods of communication.

One means of communication that people often turn to with negative results is passive-aggression. Without even knowing it, many people choose a passive-aggressive lifestyle in which they do not directly address issues that upset them but take out their frustration in unrelated ways.[1] They will try to avoid blowing things out of proportion so intently that they don't express their feelings of dissatisfaction over issues that truly bother them.

The problem is that when you avoid telling another how you feel, you tend to let it fester, which can create an inner hatred for someone. Since most of us have a hard time concealing our feelings, a person you grow to hate may pick up on your change in attitude and simply think you are being mean for no reason (because you didn't communicate your feelings to that person). So he/she may react to your hostility by acting mean toward you. This begins a cycle in which both people treat each other poorly, thinking the problems were started by the other. Over time, people come to hate each other because of issues that should have been dealt with long ago.

Passive-aggression only leads to problems. It involves repression and projection of your emotions in unbalanced ways. With passive-aggression, it is your reaction to the situation that makes things worse. Instead of speaking up, you just believe people should know how to act. The reason passive-aggression fails is because it avoids communication. The reason people do it is because it avoids confrontation.

Aggressive-Aggression

Those who rely on passive-aggression are not open about how they feel whereas others come right out and say it…loudly. Some people address others using aggression because they feel that being domineering will make others submissive to what they want. They believe that using profanity, a high yelling volume, or even physical abuse as a means to communicate their feelings is the most effective way to get others to listen and respond.

While victimizing others through aggressive communicative tactics may occasionally get you what you want, nothing comes easy. Think about how much energy you put forth by becoming aggressive. You get riled up, stressed out, and lose the ability to focus on anything besides what is bothering you. You disregard mutual respect with another person purely for the desire to get what you want.

The problem is that by disregarding respect in the effort to get what you want, you don't give others any reason to want to help you. They may still end up changing their behavior because they care, to avoid an argument, or possibly out of personal fear. But if aggression becomes habit and respect becomes evidently absent, the relationship will end; and then no amount of aggression will get it back.

Complaining

Another common and ineffective method of communication is complaining. Sometimes people complain to the person who upset them. Other times, people complain to anyone who will listen. This is occasionally referred to as venting by those who feel they need to talk about what is bothering them. But there is a big difference between discussing your feelings and condemning anyone or anything that has made your life more difficult. And sometimes, even though you think you might be expressing yourself, you're really just complaining.

Every one of your complaints is from you not getting what you want in a world in which you are judging what is right and what is wrong. Complaining causes you to focus strictly on the negative. And if you are listening to a voice say negative things about your life, no matter where that voice comes from, it will eventually make you feel bad. By complaining, you continue to remind yourself how bad your circumstances are instead of finding an effective way of moving on.

When you complain to others, people will often use the opportunity to offer you advice that could improve your circumstances. However, complaints are usually so loud in your head that they tend to block out any suggestions that someone might offer to help remedy difficulties. Realistically though, it's likely that when you complain, you're not really looking for helpful suggestions; more likely, you just want others to agree with you. You may think that if someone else confirms you have a right to be upset, you will feel better. However, even if someone agrees with you, you still have to deal with whatever you are complaining about.

The problem with complaining is that it reinforces the idea that you are a victim. Instead of focusing on what you can do to improve a situation, you focus on whomever or whatever you believe wronged you. You tell yourself that you shouldn't have to deal with the struggle, but it is your refusal to accept an experience the way it is while focusing on the difficulties it presents that makes it feel like a struggle. So complaining doesn't just make you feel bad; it keeps the bothersome situation in your life longer by distracting you from focusing on a solution.

Instead of trying to convince yourself or anyone else that you are justified in feeling bad, take action to improve your circumstances. If a car in front of you is going slow, go around it without making a big deal about it. If someone else got the promotion that you believe you earned, work harder, speak up, or find a new job. Stop blaming and start doing. I told you right from the beginning of this book that no one was going to get you through this life but you. I recognize that occasionally people make your life unnecessarily more difficult, but when you complain about it, *you* are the one making your life unnecessarily more difficult.

Persistent Thought

Have you ever had a dream where you fought with someone and when you awoke, you were upset with the person who was in your dream? The incident was in your head and, therefore, not real; but it affected your view of that person in real life, at least temporarily. These types of fictional encounters happen for many people, but many times they occur when people are awake.

Having been a persistent complainer, I know that sometimes complaining about the frustrations you encounter can feel like an involuntary reaction. It can seem almost impossible to let go of certain experiences that bother you. And when there is no one around, the complaining occurs all inside your head.

In an attempt to avoid making the same mistake twice, many people repeatedly recreate situations in their heads that they have already lived through, imagining what might have transpired had they acted differently. People also engage in fictional conversations with others based upon how they think a future dialogue might transpire. Some occasionally even go so far as to get into arguments with people—all inside their own heads. They then get upset about these imaginary experiences as though they actually occurred.

The problem with these internal conflicts is that both sides of the conversation in your head are your own voice. There is no alternative perspective to consider other than your own negative view of a situation. So your thoughts just perpetuate your feelings of frustration.

Thought is a pattern that we all rely on to survive in this world, but when you focus on problems over solutions, your thoughts can become irritations that batter you down day after day, reminding you of how bad things are. It is up to you to own situations. You need to play a conscious role in determining which thoughts you silence and which ones you let affect your mood. Either deal with a situation or let it go, but rehashing the same negative thoughts endlessly will leave you struggling for peace in your life. The only way you can move forward is by blocking out the subconscious thoughts that keep coming back to validate an opinion that is working against you. But how do you control those thoughts that seem to endlessly wonder into your head that cause you frustration? You shush them.

Technique: Shushing

When you get upset by engaging in a fictional conversation, reliving a negative experience, or complaining in your head, just say "shhh" out loud to silence your thoughts. Don't say the word "shush." Make the sound, "shhh." The sound is gentler on you and still gets the point across to your brain that what you are doing is not helping your cause of eliminating negativity from your life.

You may find yourself shushing your thoughts a lot. That is fine. You might have a pattern of subconscious negative thoughts, which you need to break. Sometimes you may get into deep conversations with someone else inside your head and realize only after getting upset that you need to shush yourself. It doesn't matter how long you've been talking to yourself or how intense a conversation in your head may get; as soon as you recognize what you are doing, shush yourself and relax.

Persistent thought is caused by having an abundance of focus. Shushing helps blind that focus so you can concentrate on other things that make you feel good. It acts as a tool for lenting by eliminating the mindless chatter in your head that isn't really focusing on a solution but self-validation of your right to complain. When you have lost control of your ability to let go of a situation to the voice of your own subconscious, shushing cuts out all rationalization and just says, "Be quiet." In that subsequent silence, which you create, is where you find the ability to let go of the negativity holding you back from enjoying your life.

Sometimes I merge this technique with the "It's Okay" technique. So I end up saying to myself, "Shhh, it's okay." It sounds just like something you say to a baby when it's crying, but that's what makes this so effective. These words calmed us all at one point in our lives, and calmness is something so desperately needed when you have depression. These words can help bring you back to the innocence and potential of the child you once were. So when you shush yourself and quiet your negative thoughts, make your next thought that pops into your head a positive one by reminding yourself that everything's going to be okay.

The negative thoughts that repeat in your head do not occur because of what has happened to you; they occur because of how you view their effect on your life. And in looking back at what caused your life to be this way, it always comes back to you because your actions have always been and are always in your control. Deep down, the real issue in every reoccurring negative thought is that had you acted differently, things might be better off now.

The results of your decisions, actions, and experiences are not always what you desire; but continually reliving a situation in which you did not succeed will repeatedly make you feel bad about your life. Other than this moment that you are living in right now, everything that has happened, could have happened, may happen, or will happen is just a thought.

Think about the situations that bother you from third-party points of view rather than having imagined arguments.

Think about the past in terms of how you acted and how another person acted rather than what you think either of you should have done. Ask yourself questions rather than asking a fictional person questions and making up the answers you think you would get in a real conversation. Explore the world rather than cursing it. Letting go of your negativity is simply letting go of your negative thoughts to enjoy the moment in which you are living.

Assertiveness

Any mathematician can tell you that the shortest distance between two points is a straight line. There are countless ineffective ways of trying to communicate with others, but the best approach is the most direct approach. That approach is assertiveness.

Being assertive means confronting a situation head on. It means that instead of tiptoeing around others' lies, actions that bother you, or perspectives you don't think are appropriate, you speak up about what you know, feel, and believe. This way, you get things off your chest so that they don't fester and lead to relationship problems down the line as can happen with passive-aggression.

If you believe someone is acting disrespectfully, let that person know. Don't be mean or threatening as that will only exacerbate the situation by putting the person you are speaking to on the defensive. Avoid sarcasm, yelling, mockery, or any other action that removes respect from the equation. Keep the tone of your voice calm but stern. You must maintain respect for the other person as well as respect for yourself by letting him/her know how you feel and that you aren't willing to be treated a certain way. And those people whom you plan to keep in your life will appreciate you enough to respect your feelings.

This does not mean that people won't be caught off guard when you speak up as most people are not used to having their actions questioned. While a few may react defensively to your assertiveness, in time most people will appreciate your candor and know they can count on your honesty. Just keep in mind which issues are worth addressing and which are worth letting go. The last thing you want is to have your assertiveness cause you to start blowing things out of proportion.

Calling people out should be done in moderation and only about issues that matter to you. Be careful not to take your assertiveness to extremes. There is a fine line between being assertive and being rude. Don't cross that line of battering people. If you spend too much of your time looking at how others can do better, two things happen: 1.) You do not grow mentally because you are critiquing others and not yourself, and 2.) You won't have any friends because people will feel as though their personalities aren't good enough for you. Assertiveness is not meant as a method to point out others' flaws but to show people that you care about your relationships with them. It's a means to open up the lines of communication, respect one another's feelings, and explore the depths of your relationships.

You are not the only one affected by other people. Those who care about you are affected by what you do and the way you feel. So if you believe that expressing your feelings to someone will take away that person's happiness, think twice about speaking up. Consider how vital it is to your own well-being that you comment on a particular issue. The core of a relationship is respect and that may occasionally mean not expressing every uncomfortable feeling you have if it is likely to take away someone's happiness. Everyone is sensitive, whether they exhibit it or not; and being direct without being sensitive to others' feelings is being insensitive.

A good rule to live by is to avoid expressing disapproval about an issue unless it is important, it directly pertains to you, or you are asked for your opinion. On the other hand, when you have positive outlooks on anything, speak up. Your encouragement is valuable to those around you, and no one likes someone who only criticizes without equally praising.

Pointing out what others do that makes you feel good can sometimes be even more effective in improving your relationships than pointing out what bothers you because it makes both you and those people feel good. For example, if you are frustrated by someone being regularly late, instead of exclusively focusing on this flaw, show your appreciation to that person anytime he/she shows up early. Your appreciation may just encourage that person to try harder to win such praise again.

Assertiveness alleviates a lot of the frustration that can often remain pent up. People will screw up at times and need to be forgiven, but sometimes people also need to apologize for their actions. If you want an apology from someone whom you're not getting one from, just ask that person for an apology. Allowing negative thoughts to stew in your mind about what you believe is right and wrong, what you think you deserve, and what you didn't get will not make situations better.

You may believe that people should realize their indiscretions on their own, but this doesn't always happen. Asking for an apology may encourage people to contemplate their actions; however, you must be prepared to likewise offer an apology as the person with whom you are being assertive may feel that you also acted inappropriately. While you may not believe you bear any responsibility, look at this type of response as an offer of insight into how your actions affect others. This is conflict, and the result is the opportunity for growth.

Part of being assertive is recognizing your role in situations. You must be willing to take what you dish out and, therefore, be willing to accept personal criticism. However, you must not purely rely on others to tell you when you have acted inappropriately. It is also *your job* to monitor your own behavior. You have a journal. When you read it, determine whether you are acting appropriately. Remember not to be mean or abrasive but maintain respect in your relationship with yourself. When you error, admit your mistake, ask forgiveness of those you may have caused harm, and document the experience in your journal.

Everyone screws up now and again, but how you deal with your mistakes is an excellent showing of whether you learned something from your actions. In fact, many people prefer those who can admit their mistakes and do better over those who were always good-natured because they serve as inspiration on how to handle personal transgressions. Regretting or denying your mistakes causes you to remain stagnant; learning from them and doing better in the future is growing up.

The Other Side of Assertiveness

Effective communication is not just about speaking but listening. Allow people to express themselves just as you want to express yourself to them. This helps avoid miscommunication as you begin to learn where everyone stands.

In some cases, however, your assertiveness will be met with silence. Some people may feel intimidated by your assertiveness or simply not know how to react. It's important to ask them to respond. Show a genuine interest in their feelings. Explain to them that the reason you are reaching out is because you care about their feelings and your relationship with them. This clarification of respect may give others the encouragement they need to open up to you.

The reason to encourage others to speak up and for you to listen to what they have to say is to help you understand them since you are the one who has the problem. If you are upset by someone else's actions, you need to find a way to move past what is bothering you. And in the effort to heal a relationship that is marred by your feelings of frustration, it helps to get down to the bottom of both what you are feeling and what another person is feeling.

When people respond, listen to what they have to say; but also consider how they say it. Just as your approach affects how well you communicate your feelings, how others present themselves to you may be representative of their feelings. If you pick up on suggestive tones, body language, or unusual reactions to you, use your assertiveness to inquire whether there are deeper issues affecting their feelings. While their approaches to you may not be suggestive of anything contrary to what they are saying, it doesn't hurt to ask.

It's essential, however, that you don't simply rely on the response you get from someone to make you feel better; the point of assertiveness is to initiate a conversation to improve your relationship. Listen to whether a person's explanation for behavior holds water and respond to that. If you don't hear the person out, you will not learn his/her point of view. This can cause you to point out the same issue repeatedly, inhibiting you both from moving on.

Showing respect for others' views and feelings will almost always lend itself to better communication than judgment. Understanding the intentions behind what people say and do can significantly help to improve the quality of your relationships. But even when assertiveness doesn't create the connections you seek, it shows you tried; and that may be the most resolution you will get.

A Letter Is Never the End

When it comes to being assertive, some people believe that they cannot say everything they want to say in person because they will be interrupted, feel intimidated, or forget what they want to say when the time comes to speak up. They may feel that writing down their feelings helps them express what they want to say. But while collecting your thoughts on paper can be incredibly helpful, it is no way to resolve issues because it avoids being direct with others.

When you write to someone without being in that person's presence, it is easier not to think about that person's feelings. For some, this makes expressing themselves easier; but the point of communication is to improve a relationship, and disregarding someone's feelings serves the opposite purpose. Emails, texts, computer postings, letters, or notes are all one-sided. They do not open up a healthy form of communication, and nothing ever gets solved this way.

Methods like texting, instant messaging, and emailing may have made our lives easier in many ways; but they can be problematic when used to address important situations. They lead to rereading messages and questioning if everything was said appropriately. They leave documentation of language you might regret and can easily be shown to others. Furthermore, they often prohibit situations from fully moving on because they can be referenced in the future.

There is also the problem that if someone doesn't respond right away to a message, the sender begins to wonder what the delay means. Was the message not received? Is the person reacting badly? Is the message being shared with others? Writing someone, which at one time may have seemed like an excellent way to communicate, can sometimes cause you more stress. As your mood changes over time, you may feel differently about what you wrote and become anxious over the endless reasons why your message did not elicit a response.

If you truly feel that a letter is the only way to get your feelings across, write down your thoughts and read them in front of the person whom you want to address. You could also hand a letter to him/her and have the person read it in front of you. This way, the other person can respond in your presence and a dialogue can unfold.

You might consider the phone to be a healthy alternative to writing a letter since there are immediate replies from those with whom you are communicating and no paper trail. However, phone calls still avoid a sense of reality. When on the phone, you can benefit by utilizing your comfort zone to speak freely without any anxious feelings. The downside unveils itself when you come in physical contact with the person. Suddenly, you don't have your comfort zone and are forced to put your words into practice, as is the other person. Had you confronted the person face to face from the start, you would have gotten this reintroduction out of the way.

The truth is that every relationship needs respect at its core, and not confronting someone directly does not show respect for that person. It also fails to display respect for you. It's important that you are able to communicate directly with the people you have relationships with because communication is an important means of displaying respect. If you can't honor your own feelings in the presence of someone else, you're best served cutting your losses and focusing on the relationships where respect does exist.

I understand, however, that on occasion writing a letter will be your only option of communicating with someone. Maybe the person is far away or refuses to talk to you. Whatever the case, if you write a letter, remember these two guidelines: 1.) Don't write anything hurtful in documentation, and 2.) Before you hit the "Send" button, post a note on a door, or mail a letter, allow your feelings to ferment.

Give yourself at least 24 hours before sending anything in writing if your intent is to address something you feel passionate about. People typically post or send messages in the heat of anger because they want to explain their points of view as quickly as possible. However, it's important to consider the various perspectives of any situation. No one stays mad all the time. Your mood will change, and you may feel differently looking back on what you wrote than the way you felt when you originally wrote a message to someone.

Different people will similarly be experiencing different emotions than you and may not always interpret what you said the same way you intended it to be understood. Letters can sometimes be misconstrued because people read them in their own tones on the heels of their own experiences. This is one reason that sarcasm typically translates so poorly in written messages. Giving yourself 24 hours to experience different emotions will give you the opportunity to think about a situation from different perspectives and better formulate your thoughts. It may seem like a long time to wait, but it's better than putting something permanently in writing based on a temporary feeling.

How you choose to communicate with others is all part of improving your relationships. It's an opportunity to understand others and be understood. And in the effort to improve the way you interact with everyone you encounter, it's up to you to be direct and respectful.

The real problem that many people have in their interactions with others is not blowing things out of proportion or ineffective communication but both in combination. Many people will actually blow little things out of proportion while not speaking up about important issues, which is the opposite of what you want to do. However, when you know what is a priority and worth your attention, you address issues with an appropriate level of intensity.

Some things in life aren't worth your attention. Sometimes those are people, and sometimes those are the ways people treat you. But when you respect yourself, you take the time to speak up about the way you feel. When you respect others, you take the time to listen to how they feel. When you are assertive with your feelings, people respect you.

The number one fear in this world is public speaking, which can easily extend to assertiveness because it involves initiating a dialogue.[2] So it is no wonder so many people avoid confrontation. However, being assertive does not necessarily mean confronting people about the inappropriate way they treat you. Being assertive is speaking up for yourself. And when you speak up about how you feel, you remind yourself and those in your life just how important the way you feel is.

Don't be afraid to be upfront with your genuineness. It's who you are. Don't be afraid to listen to how you make others feel. It's how you grow. Embrace yourself because your feelings matter and they matter to those who choose to spend time with you. When it comes to communication, you are not so much talking about issues as you are talking about your relationships.

If you never express yourself,
no one will ever know the real you.

Chapter 19

Vacationing with Anger

I'm going to tell you the story of how I became depressed, which I now understand because of the self-examination I have done. As a child, I had a fierce temper. I unleashed it often on family and friends nearly anytime I didn't get my way or felt they had ruined what I had, even if it was unintentional.

Then when I was 16 years old, I traveled overseas and realized how badly I had been acting. I decided at that point to get my temper under control. The problem was that I didn't just focus on keeping my composure; I came down on myself for how I had acted in the past. I redirected my anger, no longer visibly projecting it outward at others but privately directing it inward at myself.

I didn't forgive myself for my past, and because of that, I didn't let go of my anger. I simply found a new reason to be mad, a new person to blame for what was wrong. In this way, I let my past determine who I was. I quietly scolded myself so I would do better instead of encouraging myself, never patting myself on the back for my effort or progress. While I appeared more mature to those around me, this type of motivation was weighing heavily on my happiness. It didn't even occur to me that the reason I was feeling sad wasn't because of how I had acted in the past but because of how I was treating myself in the present.

I had lost all respect in the relationship with myself. And so my life began falling apart. I cried, I gave up, I demanded more, I got sick, and I couldn't even function at times. I hadn't felt depression before and, therefore, didn't recognize these as signs that it was coming until it was too late.

As years went by and my depression worsened, I began looking down on others as a scapegoat for my depression so that I wouldn't have to face myself. But anytime I was alone, the silence around me was filled with anxiety. I was angry. I was sad. I was lonely. I had no closure with my past and no appreciation of my present. Everything meant something deep to me, and with a negative perspective, everything meant something bad about my life. Everyone at some point seemed like an enemy. I felt surrounded by a world of negativity, measuring a good day by what didn't go wrong.

Then one beautiful spring day, I sat in my apartment and thought about my life with a mouth full of pills. I felt I had lost everything that mattered, and it seemed to make sense that I might as well give up my life as well. All I had to do was swallow, and that would be it. Such a simple act—a simple act that I never went through with for the simple fact that I didn't really want to die. I wanted the pain to go away so badly, but what I wanted was a happy life, not the end of my life.

That was the day I almost gave up my life, but the way I remember it is as the day that I didn't give up my life. There were so many moments after that day in which I questioned whether to finish the job. Every time someone criticized me or gave up on me, I felt like giving up too. But there were a few people who believed in me, and I eventually became one of them. I learned to stand up for myself.

Over the next three and a half years, I dedicated my life to learning about myself, this world, and how we interact with each other. I gathered my thoughts, my realizations, and my experiences; and I put them down on paper. And in that course study of life, I finally began to understand my anger, my depression, and how they were related.

For many people who are depressed or on the verge of depression, anger comes easily and often. Getting angry provides a feeling of power when someone or something gets in the way of you having the life you want. It makes you believe that you are above others who have somehow wronged you, but anger is really just a veil for a different emotion.

Taking a close look at anger involves exploring its relationship to sadness. When you get mad, something bigger is going on than the fact that you are not getting your way. The truth is that you get mad because you are sad. Perhaps you feel that someone hurt you, or maybe it is because of how you handled a situation. You turn to anger as a replacement for sadness because it gives you breathing room from the sorrow in your life.

Anger feels like a burst of energy, which is exactly what you need to motivate yourself to improve your life. Sadness, on the other hand, feels like your energy is being drained as you focus on how your pain feels. Therefore, just like taking a vacation to avoid your regular routine, anger helps you to vacation from your sadness by providing you energy and changing your focus from the pain you feel to who is at fault for causing your pain. But all vacations must come to an end, and similarly, you must find ways other than being mad to live well.

While anger is an effective way to take your focus off your sadness, its effect is only temporary. Anger doesn't get rid of your pain; it merely diverts your focus while providing you energy, which you can then use toward creating a better life for yourself. However, if you don't use that energy to make improvements to your overall life, you will feel the pain of sadness anytime you're not angry. This can cause many people to become addicted to anger as a means of continually hiding their sadness since that is easier than making genuine improvements.

When anger takes over your life, you get wrapped up in the blame game. You remove any responsibility for having caused your circumstances or any feeling that you are responsible for resolving them. Instead, you criticize anyone or anything that you feel caused you to feel bad, be it loved ones, strangers, or God. You condemn them in order to invalidate what they have done to you in an effort to invalidate your pain, but blaming others never makes your pain go away permanently.

The real reason you so quickly turn to blaming others is not so much because they caused you to feel bad but because you already felt bad. Whether you want to admit it or not, your perception was that your life was not going well, only now you have an excuse for why. You may believe that your life was good before certain incidents took place, but if you were truly happy, you wouldn't allow another's actions to shake your world so much. You'd simply realize that your problems could be handled by the strengths that exist in your life.

The energy that anger provides you can feel freeing from your sadness, but energy is meant to be used and exchanged for new energy. Your anger exists to help you overcome harmful circumstances and move on. Too often though, anger's energy is used to harm those you feel have harmed you. And in that aggression, you don't move on but rather hold on to the sadness in your life that is being veiled by your own anger.

Revenge Is an Endless Battle

Sadness can immobilize you during depression, but when you start embracing anger, you take the focus off your sadness. Lifting this weight from your shoulders will provide a substantial amount of energy, and you will want to use it. When people get angry, they often want to lash out. They want to shout, take revenge, and destroy any cause of their suffering. Instead of focusing on how they are hurt, they focus on wanting to hurt another. They want their influences to feel the suffering that they have felt.

With revenge, you almost feel like it is both your duty and your right to get back at someone who has made you feel bad. The reason you typically feel this way is because you believe the person who caused you harm is in some way better off than you. You feel weak and revenge can seem like an effective way to take control of the situation. You believe that taking away someone's happiness who took away yours will validate your strength and even the playing field, but the problem is that bringing someone down doesn't bring you up. Many believe that the principle of "an eye for an eye" is justified, but Mahatma Gandhi may have been right when he said that taking "an eye for an eye makes the whole world blind."[1] I subscribe to Gandhi's perspective because revenge blinds you from yourself. It stifles your ability to move on. It keeps your focus outward.

Getting mad and demanding retribution will only cause an unfortunate situation to go on longer than it should. You will stew in your misery, demand justice, and be angry until you feel the person who upset you has sufficiently paid for his/her wrongdoing. Your desire for revenge will also typically be more hurtful or intense than the action originally committed against you because what you are truly seeking in revenge is for justice to put your pain to rest.

The truth is that there is no amount of suffering by another that will ease your pain, making revenge an endless battle. Many people who lose someone to murder and then are able to witness the murderer be executed do not feel better afterward. In fact, they often feel worse. They have taken on the role of the hater. They have brought themselves down to the level of the person who wronged them. They have focused on increasing another's pain instead of healing their own pain, and it led them to a worse place. With anger, it's easy to believe that justice equals closure; but there is no grieving in revenge. There is only more hatred and the festering of an already bad situation.

You may believe that certain people ought to be punished for their actions, but trying to punish them yourself requires a lot of energy, a lot of attention, and a lot of time. Every moment that you focus on punishing the cause of your pain, you are focusing on your pain, which only makes you feel worse about your life. It's like getting hurt twice except you're intentionally causing it the second time.

While things may seem bad in the heat of the moment, revenge can severely exacerbate your circumstances.

Depending on how vengeful you want to be, you risk getting arrested or encouraging the person you are trying to hurt to attack you in retaliation. You create an environment for yourself in which you risk what you have for someone you don't care about.

There is always the possibility of committing an act of vengeance against another person and not getting caught. While at a glance, this might seem like the perfect solution, it causes the situation to linger for the rest of your life. If you get away with revenge, you live with the indefinite possibility of getting caught for your action. You are forced to keep what you've done hidden for the rest of your life. You will never be able to fully open up to anyone, making your life a vault that you have to guard forever.

On top of all this, committing revenge against another may lead to good things happening for the person you hurt. Just as you charted in your journal how difficult experiences in your life have opened up opportunities for you over time, the same is true for everyone. This means that if you do something mean to someone, your action may lead to something great for that person that he/she otherwise would not have enjoyed. In an attempt to commit revenge, you will likely help that person out, which might make you angrier.

Revenge is a symptom of having an abundance of focus, and because of that, it can overtake your thinking. Even the personal debate over whether to commit revenge can supersede anything else that requires your attention. You have to determine for yourself how much you are willing to let the past impact your life now and whether it will determine the course of your future. What has transpired doesn't have to hold as much weight as you may believe it does. I know how much it can hurt. I know what it feels like to wake up every morning feeling sad and know the reason, but punishing the cause of your pain is not going to make your pain go away because it won't change what has happened to you. Your focus and effort must continuously be to better yourself, not to wrong another.

You will discover that the moment after you decide not to commit vengeance against another, you release an exhaustive breath that relieves a significant amount of negativity from your life. You instantly open up the opportunity to focus on improving the way you feel instead of trying to play God. When you come to the conclusion not to harm another, you no longer have to worry about the possibility of retaliation for your action, the possibility of getting caught, or the energy revenge would require of you. You instead get to be a good person and can be proud of the way you live your life.

Finding pleasure in someone else's pain has no long-term benefits. You don't need to embrace others' indirect encouragement for you to be mean when you really want to be a good person. You'll end up hating people for making you feel bad and hating yourself for how you've acted.

Confronting the Issue

Getting angry gives you space from your sadness, but it doesn't give you peace of mind. Anger is not meant to be kept in your life indefinitely. It is a tool, not a solution. To truly let go of the anger in your life, you must eliminate the sadness; and that means healing your pain.

When you use anger to handle conflicts in your life that have been brought on by someone else, you're best served addressing the person and situation assertively. Rather than projecting your anger at another, confront that person; and ask everything you want to know. This way, you gain clarity about your circumstances; and understanding precedes acceptance and your ability to move on.

You may not get all the answers you want or even your questions answered at all, but if you don't try, you may always wonder. Using your assertiveness, say everything that you want to say as well; but be genuine. Make sure to keep your tone even and your volume low, and avoid cursing. Remember that being assertive doesn't mean being cruel.

The real issue when you are upset, however, is not what happened but how what happened makes you feel. For example, if someone lied to you, is the issue really that he/she lied or is it that you feel like your trust was abused? If your lover is spending a lot of time with someone else, is the issue really the time spent with another or that you are afraid of losing the person you love from your life? Rather than focusing on the details of a situation (which are just results), take the time to understand and discuss the underlying issue: what it is about a situation that makes you upset and why. And when it comes to your anger, your underlying feelings are always related to something that makes you feel sad.

If you disregard the underlying issue and only focus on the specific circumstances at hand, any resolution you come to will only be temporary. When different circumstances later arise, the same conversation may unfold because you didn't address the real issue affecting your feelings; you only addressed the incident. This is a key reason why people often feel like they have the same arguments repeatedly. They never focus on what is guiding their feelings about the actions that lead into arguments.

Focusing on the ins and outs of problems are the subtopics of your feelings. You don't need to know the details of a situation to know how you feel; you only need to know yourself. When you understand where your feelings are coming from, you can better assess whether they are based on beliefs that can be compromised or should stay intact.

Anytime yelling, interruptions, or violence enter a conversation, it's time to reconsider your approach because respect has been lost: respect for how the other person should be spoken to and respect for yourself to address what is actually guiding your feelings. Anger plays an important role in your life, but its purpose is not for communication. When anger causes communication to break down, use that break to let moods change and emotions calm.

Technique: Calming Down

I've discussed in this book how the body and mind are connected and that you can use one to affect the other. Well, one of the best and simplest ways I have found to reduce momentary feelings of anger is to pay attention to how you are posing your body. When angry, many people will cross their arms, thereby creating a barrier between themselves and others because they are on the defensive. Other times, they might use their torso and hand gestures to project themselves forward because they are on the offensive. In both cases, their shoulders are lurching forward, forcing all their energy outward and blocking themselves off from anything getting in. Essentially, they are taking on a fighting stance.

But in an effort to calm yourself, you must give up the fight both mentally and physically. Instead of crossing your arms or forcing all your energy outward, you must take the opposite stance.

Place both hands behind your back with one hand gently clasping the wrist of the other hand. Make sure to roll your shoulders back when you take this posture. When you hold these parts of your body back, you also hold back the anger that you feel. The posture literally stretches out your torso, opening you up and making you feel better both physically and mentally.

Just as you may have seen old wise men in films walking with their arms behind their backs, this physical action relaxes the anger of the mind. By similarly going for a walk outside while holding this posture, you expose yourself to fresh air, release any pent up energy through exercise, and give yourself physical space to complement the mental space you are taking so that you can rationally think about what is frustrating you.

———

Eliminating Your Trigger

Sometimes anger is not a momentary event. Occasionally those who have upset you can have such an effect on your life that you get upset by the mere presence of them. Those you blame for causing you harm are your *triggers* because they cause you to lose control of your emotions. They are the salt to your wound, and that means that you must eliminate them from your life until that wound is healed so that they are no longer triggers but merely a part of your journey through life.

Wounds often need space to heal, and when your anger does not die down by confronting someone else assertively, you must take space from your trigger to truly heal. This is important because if you just used anger to minimize your sadness but continued to focus on what bothered you, you would only intensify your anger.

You may think that taking space from your trigger would be ignoring a situation, but that is hardly the case. Ignoring something means not worrying about it because you deem it insignificant. Taking space, on the other hand, requires a conscious effort to abstain from engaging whatever is influencing your emotional turmoil. It is not simply the experience of being separated from your trigger that makes a difference; taking space means that *you* are the one creating distance. *You* are the one who is walking away. If space between you and someone is forced upon you but you remain focused on your trigger, you will never heal. Your focus needs to be on you and your own growth. So even if you are not the one to initially create space, once you decide to be an enforcer of that space in order to focus on your own healing, you gain control of your space.

In a way, taking space is a lot like lenting. It separates you from a single focus so that you can begin appreciating what you're disregarding and realize that you don't need everything you're focusing on. When you take space for yourself, you gain a new perspective that is no longer guided significantly by circumstances that have upset you.

It is important that once you decide to avoid your trigger, you do it. Your mood will change as will your realizations. But if you engage someone—one moment acting nice, another moment acting mad, and yet another moment acting needy— you will turn into the person causing problems.

Earlier in this book, I discussed looking at negative situational patterns as "Lucy" from the "Peanuts" comic strip. While "Lucy" is an appropriate label for anything that repeatedly entices you into something that causes you pain, when you get uncontrollably angry around a particular person, you may need to treat that person like "Medusa."

Medusa in Greek mythology was a character that upon looking at, people would turn to stone.[2] Well, consider that when you are around a person that helps fuel your anger, you are unable to move on. You become stuck as though you were turned to stone. And the more you focus on your trigger, the angrier you become, solidifying the feeling of immobility more and more in your life.

The reason the person causing you pain has taken on the label of Medusa is not because the person is causing you trouble every moment of every day. The person has taken on this label because of how you are affected by him/her. "Lucy" is how the person is acting; "Medusa" is how the person affects you. This means that even when someone who caused you pain is not presently hurting you, you may still be angry at how the person acted in the past. In order to avoid feeling bad, you must, therefore, avoid what is triggering your unhappiness; and that means separating yourself from the person you associate with a painful time in your life.

When taking space from someone, you must do your best to avoid the person both in the outside world and in your head. Avoid talking about the person, looking for the person, inquiring what the person is doing with his/her life, or investigating whether the person has spoken about you if it only makes you angry. You may need to stop going to places where you will be forced to see someone that makes you feel uncomfortable. You may need to take a break from social networking websites like "Facebook," "LinkedIn," or the dating site where you may have met someone if you end up searching for that person only to get upset. It may even help to remove items from your home if they keep reminding you of someone or a situation that is making you feel bad. Whatever makes you angry (causes you to turn to stone) should be avoided.

Utilizing the "Shushing" technique from the last chapter can help to control those compulsive thoughts in your head that create an abundance of focus on another. The world may be a big place, but there are many things you can do to make it feel quite small. Use your anger for space. In a civilized world, that is its purpose. You need to learn to live for yourself, not for another person.

Rearranging your life may seem unfair, but remember that taking space is for your own well-being. Only you can determine how much space you need based on your reaction to your trigger. If you give up the space you need because you are overly focused on what you want, you risk causing yourself continued aggravation. The separation you must take is temporary yet important to give to yourself until your trigger no longer has control over your emotional state. You should be the one to decide whether you remain angry.

Reactions

It's important to know that taking space from people can have a profound effect *on them*. There are three possible reactions that those you take space from will display. The first possible reaction is that someone you are avoiding will begin seeking your attention through kindness. The person may recognize how much his/her actions hurt you and not want to lose you from his/her life. The person may even apologize and try to spend time together with you.

Reactions of kindness are typically brief, and if you want to take advantage of them, you must do this when you first encounter them because it will probably be the only time they happen. People often want what they can't have, and your avoidance of someone suggests to that person that he/she cannot have your affection. Hence, the person desires it. If you receive an apology, acknowledge and accept it; however, if you are still angry and unable to move on, do not welcome the person back into your life yet. The other person can't just be ready to move on; you must be ready too.

When someone is nice to you, it's important to understand exactly what that person's kindness means. Many people who have been hurt by those they love (particularly those with whom they are infatuated) will often want to embrace any interest they receive. This can often lead to confusion about what having those people back in their lives means. It is your assertiveness that will allow you to question what someone is looking for in a relationship beyond a solitary act of kindness.

Otherwise, there is the potential for misunderstanding and further personal disappointment.

The second reaction you may encounter when you avoid people is that they will try to affect your life through negative means. This can happen because the person you are taking space from may believe your avoidance is a form of attack. Or that person might want your attention and not know how to accomplish that. So he/she may attempt to cause you harm so that you pay attention to him/her. Whatever the reason, if someone launches an attack on you for taking space, you must continue to avoid the person. Just like giving in to a child who cries for attention, if you give in to a person's inappropriate behavior, you are essentially telling the person that acting mean to you will get your attention.

It's also important to keep your distance in the face of negative attacks because of *your* needs. If you were angry enough that you needed separation from someone, after a new display of negativity toward you, direct engagement will only result in you losing control of your emotions. And you shouldn't give up what you are working toward for someone who is being mean. You took time to yourself for a reason. This is an example of your commitment to yourself being tested.

If the negative circumstances being thrust upon you go overboard, you may need to speak to friends of that person or turn to legal channels. You will need to determine the threat level you are encountering and what type of response is necessary based on that.

Occasionally your interactions with one person will become bigger than the two of you. One method of gaining your attention through negative means may include the involvement of others. The person you are avoiding may use the space you are taking to encourage people to dislike you. These will typically be close friends of the person you are avoiding and appear to them as simply friends discussing one another's lives even though there may be an ulterior motive. The person you are avoiding may realize his/her actions were inappropriate and make an effort to convince others that his/her behavior was actually justified.

When someone has brought outsiders into personal dilemmas, you will find yourself left with the decision of whether to stand up for yourself and explain your position or to remain silent in order for the drama to fade away. Unfortunately, this can very easily become a lose-lose situation. Allow me to elaborate.

You often hear that first impressions are lasting ones. Well, consider that the first time people hear about a specific issue is their first impression of it. Rarely do they consider that there could be an alternative truth. They typically assume that the person telling the story is just bringing their attention to an issue and naturally accept what they are told at face value.

If you stand up against gossip being spread about you, people tend to feel that you are pressuring them to choose sides. By giving them an alternative reality to consider, they would likely become upset with you or simply not believe you. You would be forcing them to reexamine what they know. You would be forcing them to embrace the possibility of change, and many people unfortunately oppose that.

On the other hand, if you don't say anything in your defense, you will not get yourself into more trouble; but others will assume you have something to hide and are, therefore, the problem. They will think everything they hear from one source is true, never considering that it might be skewed in its truth. So understandably, you cannot successfully utilize either of these options.

Your opportunity will be to open people's minds to the real truth or at least a different perspective. Your intention should not be to bring others to your side but to paint an accurate picture. The best way to deal with a contentious matter is to address the situation in small doses. People are rarely in the mood for long stories, and they don't want to know the ins and outs of someone else's relationship. They just want to know who is right and who is wrong.

Keep your defenses short and simple for the benefit of both others and yourself. Remember, if you are taking space for yourself, you are still emotionally distraught over the situation. And if you don't give yourself emotional space when you need it, any negativity that has been spread about you will be confirmed because you have yet to gain control of your emotions. However, if you take the space you need, you will be able to defend yourself rationally once you have healed, displaying your maturity and growth. And on a long enough timeline, the truth always comes out.

Actions speak louder than words, and over time, people recognize the difference between what they hear and what they witness. By living morally and being assertive when rational, many people who at one time turned against you may eventually come to reexamine their positions.

Your decision to act rationally and with kindness will be what defines you in the long run, not what people say about you. The people in this world who take the time to get to know you are the ones worth your time. Their appreciation and recognition of who you are grows from how you choose to live your life.

You will still find that some people will treat you unfairly and not be interested in what you have to say. When certain people reject you based on the one-sided commentary of another, it will prove to be their loss and your gain. Those people who let one person's negative viewpoint color their own opinion about you will lose having an amazing person in their lives, and you will avoid having people in your life who are willing to judge others based on hearsay.

Many people assume that everyone they know is a friend, but that is not always true; it often takes harsh circumstances to prove the significance of those relationships. When you encounter hard times, look around and see who cares about your feelings; and appreciate those people. Don't expect that everyone will be there for you all the time and don't get mad at those who aren't. Just appreciate the ones who prove their friendship.

Be aware that not everyone who is your friend will stand by your every decision, but every one of your friends should always keep an open mind when presented with contentious situations. You really don't want friends to blindly take your side anyway because they will just as easily take someone else's side when the next situation arises. Those who are open-minded, however, will help you to see your strengths and flaws, giving you valuable insight to grow into a better person over time.

This is an important realization because you may find it difficult to accept friends who embrace someone that you feel hurt you. You may believe that the person should not be embraced and feel that an acceptance of someone causing you pain signifies a rejection of you. However, it's typically not a rejection at all. It's more often because many people do not overwhelmingly concern themselves with anything unless it affects them directly.

Furthermore, different people have different types of relationships with those whom you might not get along with. For example, you may have a bad relationship with an ex-lover; but someone else may not be seeking a loving relationship with that person. He/she may simply want to have a beer with your ex-lover. Other people may not be concerned with whether the person you dislike is a good boyfriend/girlfriend since they simply want to socially spend time together. Their relationships with that person may have nothing to do with you even though your relationship with that person is tarnished.

When you take space for yourself, the reaction from others can bring kindness or cruelty; but there is a third response: no reaction at all. Your avoidance may not seem to affect the person you are avoiding, which might make you feel like your pain doesn't matter to that person. You may see this lack of a reaction as a reason to feel more pain, but both negative and indifferent reactions are really just proof that you made the right decision to take space. They are confirmation that you weren't getting respect.

The reality, however, is that if you avoid someone long enough, eventually that person will stop caring about your avoidance. Over time, people learn to live with their lives as they are; and that includes your absence. This is why it is so important that you never avoid someone for a reaction just as you should not be living for results.

The possible reactions you may receive from others by taking space for yourself give you valuable insight into how specific people relate to you. But what is even more important than that is what you learn about how you relate to the rest of the world. Taking space gives you a break from what is bothering you to reestablish working relationships with everything and everyone you may have disregarded. And in your lenting, you rediscover your life: what matters and what doesn't.

Letting Go of Anger

Avoiding someone is not an action that will resolve a difficult situation. It is an action that gives you breathing room until you are prepared to address the situation rationally. And so it is essential that you use the space you take to learn about your life. While staying angry may help you avoid facing your sadness, it doesn't make it go away. In time, you end up losing the confidence in yourself to handle whatever difficulties come your way. You blame, waiting for someone else to fix your life; but no one can fully alleviate the pain of past experiences except you.

Your time apart from your trigger is meant to help you calm down from the emotional upheaval of a negative experience, but it is also to define the roles of the various aspects of the experience. Through your space, you will need to recognize that your trigger is not the person who caused your frustration and sadness. The trigger is the experience. The cause is your reaction. And the results are your feelings.

Technique: Trading Anger for Appreciation

Space provides you a place to reflect, and within that space, there are three important tasks you need to commit to doing:

1.) The first and most important task is to take the time to learn about yourself. Think about how your anger might have been a shield for how you were hurt. Learn about the role you played in the relationship gone awry. Consider why your anger lingered long after the event was over. Determine whether you still want what you once did. Use the "Questions" technique from Chapter 6 to go deep.

2.) The next task is to look for connections between yourself and the person you feel harmed you. Discovering connections between you and your adversaries is essential to understanding and accepting them. Without connections, you forget that there is so much more than an incident that makes people who they are. And when you define a person by a single action that bothers you, you will subsequently feel pain as long as that person is alive.

Now you will likely want to avoid acknowledging connections between you and anyone who has harmed you. This is because when we feel that others have caused us harm, we tend to look at ourselves as innocent and the other people as guilty; and it's difficult to acknowledge good qualities in those who are guilty. Therefore, I recommend that you focus on the error in your own ways. *Don't look* for positive connections between you and the person who wronged you; look for negative ones. No one is perfect. We have all suffered at the hands of others and caused pain for those in our lives. The best way to create a connection with someone else when you are upset with that person is to recognize that you have also wronged people, whether intentionally or not.

The connection that you find with someone may not be the connection that the person recognizes with you. The person may not even acknowledge a connection with you, but in your time of space, you are the one who needs to find similarities between you and that person because you are the one in pain. When you can see how you are both alike, your anger no longer seems so important to your healing; and then you can begin to focus more on what's on the horizon rather than what's behind you.

3.) The last task you have during your separation time is to figure out how what you are angry about may actually have been what was best for you. You don't need to convince yourself that your experience was entirely positive. It's important to recognize why what happened was so bad that you felt you needed separation to control your anger about it, but it's also necessary to see the benefits it offers. Being rational means being able to see both the good and the bad in anything and accepting it for exactly what it is.

When you get angry, your anger is over a difficult experience. Open your journal and turn to the diagram you created of bad experiences that led to good experiences in your life. Then write down your hardship in the column of bad experiences on that diagram. At some point, you will be able to connect it with good experiences in your life. You may even recognize a few now. If nothing else, you might recognize that the bad experience allowed you to learn about yourself and grow as a person. And that is an advantage, which will help you for the rest of your life.

———

Using space to learn about yourself, exploring connections between you and your adversaries, and recognizing the benefits that come from hardship are keys to letting go of your anger. Without this process, you will end up holding grudges, feeling tension in the presence of others, and doubting the sincerity of those around you. These tasks may not always improve your relationships with those who have wronged you, but they allow you to be okay with what you have experienced. And sometimes that's the most you can ask for. Sometimes that's everything.

Seeking Closure
Anger is the easiest way to temporarily halt the paralyzing effects of depression, but alone, it won't allow you to overcome it. You must let go of anger to fully move on with your life. Once you are accepting of your past and comfortable in the presence of someone from whom you have taken space, prove that you have moved on by seeking closure with that person to address any unresolved issues. Avoiding dealing with the situation may be easier, but as long as you are avoiding

people, there will remain a feeling of hostility and discomfort whenever you are around, think about, or hear about them. Using your anger properly is about learning to live without people in your life the way you want them to be or learning how to live with people in your life in a way different than you want them to be. Rather than searching for a world that doesn't exist, your anger must be used as a space to accept things the way they are so that you can confront people and move on.

When you do confront others, they may be taken off guard by your interest in discussion. If someone you previously avoided questions the purpose of talking, explain your desire to move on. Offer locations for discussion that are non-threatening and free from distractions. Open spaces like parks or coffee shops allow the opportunity for either person to feel safe and free to leave if the situation becomes uncomfortable. Avoid locations that are loud and difficult to hear or where either of you are likely to be intoxicated. Don't meet at your or the other person's home or in a place filled with people either of you know who could interrupt your discussion. The point is to create an atmosphere that offers comfort and the ability to discuss feelings openly so that everyone can move on without further tension.

Use the opportunity you create to address the situation that led to your anger. Discuss how it made you feel, why it made you feel that way, and how you feel now. Then forgive that person.

Once you open up about your feelings, encourage the other person to share his/her own thoughts and feelings. Listen closely to what the person says. Answer any questions candidly and consider any validity to comments that may help you learn about yourself. If the person is frustrated with you, offer an apology and ask forgiveness. Remember, the conversation is meant to create closure, not debate who is at fault. Asking forgiveness is one of the most humbling things a human can do. It shows compassion and understanding, which is essential for closure. Both you and the other person must accept that neither of you acted completely appropriately in the situation in question.

Allowing someone else to fully accept fault is an act of revenge. You don't want the person you are seeking closure with to look back and feel bad. That isn't closure. Closure means that both you and the other person are okay with what happened and as things are now. If either person still feels bad, your relationship with each other will continue to be based on what happened. The past is over. By letting go of its attachment, everyone can move on, remembering what happened and why everyone is capable of doing better.

You must understand, however, that the person with whom you seek closure may not be ready to talk with you. Not everyone is on the same timeline as you, and you have to accept this possibility. If that person isn't willing to meet with you or let go of the past, accept that you tried and let that be enough. You took space to heal and then tried to make amends with someone whom you felt hurt you. You don't personally need closure with someone else to move on, but you do need closure with yourself to move beyond the past. And *seeking* closure with others is how you prove to yourself that you're ready to move on. Your effort is always what matters.

If someone with whom you seek closure is not ready to move on, do not feel bad for taking your separation time. It was necessary for you to secure your happiness, and now the other person may also require space. If you don't give that person the opportunity to take space, he/she will take it anyway—just like you did. And then you might think it is solely because of you even though taking space is something people do purely for themselves.

On the road to forgiveness, you cannot wait around for others to forgive you. They, like you, must find solace in their own ability to forgive because what forgiveness really means is moving on. And so when it comes to letting go of anger, seeking closure doesn't just mean forgiving others; it means forgiving yourself.

When you're angry, the person you really feel let you down is you. You are upset with your life, and that means you are truly the only one who can change it. Until you make amends with yourself, you'll continue to carry around your past, the pain it caused you, and the anger you've used to veil your sadness. Right now is an opportunity to move on to a better moment. And when you forgive yourself, you let go of what happened and the anger you no longer need. That's how you give closure to the sadness behind your anger.

There is no appreciation in anger. There is only space. It separates you from everything around you. It creates distance between you and everything bad as well as everything good. Sometimes you need this space to grow, but the point of anger is to use it and let it go.

When you keep anger in your life and look at the world, you see what is wrong with it. You see what is unfair. You see what is unjust. You see only what needs improvement. You let the bad that you see corrupt the good that exists until you forget how much good there is in this world.

When you get angry all the time, you've missed the point of anger; you've missed the opportunity in anger. Take the time to consider whether the world really is as bad as you perceive it to be or if your anger at others is just part of an attempt to avoid facing yourself.

At some point, like I did, you may have gotten angry and never let it go. And as that anger got pointed in all directions, you unavoidably got upset with yourself too. Over time, you may have fought yourself for the mistakes you made, the things you gave up too soon, what you lost, and the overall way you lived. And by not letting go of that anger, it may have taken over your life until nothing was the way you wanted it to be, possibly causing you to feel as though there was nothing left to live for.

But the space that you must take when you are angry is not about giving up everything you have; it's about changing the way you live. When you take a break from your normal day-to-day life, you begin breaking your patterns, including the pattern that involves directing your anger at yourself. As you explore your life and accept yourself as you are, there can no longer be any anger. There can no longer be any rejection. There is only opportunity as you stand up for your life by bettering yourself, not belittling yourself.

When you are exhausted from fighting, you just want to give up. But rather than giving up what matters, give up your anger by focusing on what is really behind it: an inner sadness that needs closure. The pain in your life is tough to face, but out of respect for yourself, it's time to address it and move on.

Sometimes we just need to take
a step back to appreciate what we have.

Chapter 20

Taking Responsibility

Your circumstances don't determine your life; you do. Everything you have in your life is in some way because of your doing. You weren't just given things. Your belongings, jobs, friends, and enemies are all the result of the type of person you are. It's not mere coincidence. Everything good and everything bad you possess and experience is tied to the life you have chosen to live.

Too often people blame others for negative circumstances in their lives. They look outside themselves at what is causing them to feel bad rather than recognizing their own responsibility in having caused or fixing adverse situations. They shed their responsibility because they want to believe that their actions demonstrate that they are good people even when bad things happen to them. What is problematic, however, is not their desire to be good people but denying responsibility for what transpires in their lives. It's problematic because taking responsibility is one of the best ways to take control of your life.

When something is out of your hands, like what other people do with their lives, your response can only be to find ways to deal with their behavior. But when something is your fault, you are responsible for what has happened and are, therefore, also responsible for correcting the situation. By taking action to correct the situation, you become an active participant in creating a resolution rather than being a passive observer, accepting or lamenting the negativity of the situation.

Let's say that you viewed a situation as not your fault. Another way of saying this is that you had no control over the situation. Consider what a loss that is to be at the mercy of what life throws at you. My encouragement of taking even a modest amount of responsibility for what happens in your life is because responsibility represents control. It makes your life one that you can create however you see fit.

Even in cases where others seem to hold obvious fault, the fastest way to take control of a situation that is bothering you is to take personal responsibility. Imagine a situation in which someone deliberately hurt you. By accepting the possibility that the way you have lived your life made that person want to hurt you, it becomes easier to accept the situation, forgive the person, and move on. It may not seem that your actions and the other person's actions were proportional, but the idea that you somehow played a role in causing an undesirable situation gives you a reason for what happened. And for so many people, it is not knowing why something happened that plagues their lives.

If your options for why you feel bad in relation to negative experiences are 1.) Feeling bad because something happened or 2.) Feeling bad because you caused something to happen, this second option allows you to examine yourself more. You begin to learn what behavior might have led to unfortunate circumstances and your subsequent discontent. And that understanding gives you the ability to affect the impact of what happened to you and to prevent it from happening again. Taking responsibility allows you to grow and alter your behavior to better influence what you experience. It is the essence of how you change your patterns.

When all things seem to be going wrong or you are repeatedly encountering the same type of bad experiences, you have to ask yourself whether it is just bad luck or if you have some responsibility for your detriments. I'm going to tell you a little secret: you always bear some responsibility for the circumstances you encounter—occasionally in causing your predicaments and always in how you respond to them.

Now I realize that many might look at what I am saying and suggest the opposite: that people are not always responsible for what happens to them. "What about incidents of abuse or rape?" they might say. When I suggest that people are responsible for their own experiences, I am not saying that those people did anything wrong. Nor am I saying that they are responsible for anyone's actions other than their own. However, each of us plays a key role in every one of our experiences.

If you found yourself the victim of abuse, you may not have caused someone to harm you; but how you let it affect you now *is* your responsibility. There are plenty of situations in your life in which others hold fault. And while it might seem like it is their responsibility to correct the situations, they don't always do that. Sometimes people won't even apologize. And if you are dependent on others correcting their mistakes and indiscretions for you to feel alright, you will never find peace in your life. You will spend every day demanding, complaining, and waiting for others to make life better for you.

When you recognize your role in causing yourself to feel the way you do, you become equally responsible to do something about those feelings. Taking responsibility gives you power while blaming, holding grudges, and complaining makes you a victim at the mercy of those who have wronged you. Take your life back from others. It's yours to live.

You might believe that there are some situations in which you can only blame God or nature for what is wrong, such as natural disasters, accidents, or when you or someone else gets sick. However, the results are the same if you look out to blame instead of looking in at how to move forward. It's a fact that many doctors consider depression an illness, but in reading this book, you have taken responsibility for your depression. You have looked into your life for patterns, perspectives, and approaches that are aiding your depression. You have witnessed the relationship between what you do and what you experience. And in this relationship, you can clearly see a level of control. What you have done so far in accordance with this book has given you control over your life, and you will maintain that control as long as you continue to take responsibility for your life and make an effort to keep improving it.

Technique: How to Take Responsibility

So how do you change a perspective of blaming others for your problems to claiming responsibility for your experiences? It's all in how you word your perspective. So let's review the possible ways you might describe your experiences and the role you play in each perspective.

When you first consider the reasoning behind your feelings, you likely look to obvious causes. In describing why you feel bad, you might say something like, *"That person hurt me."* Of course, this is blaming; and it only serves to make you a victim while giving all the power in your life over to the one who hurt you.

So now you might avoid giving power to the person and reword your perspective to say, *"I feel that I was wronged."* This gives no power to a specific person, but it still implies that you are not at fault and that it is someone else's responsibility to make you feel better.

Taking this another step forward by focusing exclusively on how you feel, you might articulate your perspective by saying, *"I feel betrayed"* or *"I feel hurt."* This language is better than previously worded perspectives because it concentrates on how you feel without giving away control. However, only focusing on your pain will intensify it. It does nothing to heal your wounds.

Taking responsibility means acknowledging how your own behavior affects your feelings. It means saying something like, *"I got my ego bruised"* or *"I let someone treat me a certain way."* These types of statements acknowledge that you are not responsible for the actions of others, but they also admit that you had control over your destiny because you were responsible for yourself and your feelings. You did not hurt yourself, but you allowed yourself to get hurt. You might still be sad, but there is room to grow from this mentality because you admit a mistake. And you can only make a mistake if you were in control of your own actions. Having the control to affect what happens to you as well as how you respond gives you the power to control every one of your experiences.

———

Whenever you find yourself struggling with an issue, ask yourself what is the reason. Your response will go something like this: "I am having a hard time because _____." Whatever you fill in the blank with, ask yourself whether it is the real reason for your struggle or just an excuse. The truth is that no one thing affects everything. Many factors cause you to struggle, and it's a good idea to consider whether your biggest cause of struggle is each excuse you make for why you aren't who or where you want to be. Many circumstances outside yourself will affect your life, which no one reason will explain. But every reason you do or don't do something is an excuse unless the reason is you.

For example, you may say that you don't want to go outside because it is raining; but the real reason might be because you don't want to get wet. Rather than blaming the rain for ruining the day, what is actually determining your decision not to go outside is your opinion of getting wet. Taking responsibility makes a situation better because you understand the logic guiding your feelings. You recognize what your true concern is, and from there, you can find ways to alleviate that concern. By bringing an umbrella or wearing a rain jacket, you could address what is really bothering you and take measures to eliminate the negativity of the situation.

When you view your life a certain way, you feel a certain way. This technique on how to take responsibility describes a number of different perspectives that people often use to characterize their negative experiences, but only one of them displays responsibility. When you can physically say out loud the way you feel and give yourself credit for your experiences, there becomes just one person responsible for where you go from here: you.

Whose Responsibility Is Your Responsibility?

Your life is in your hands. You are in control of it, and you are responsible for what you do with it. However, it is the only life you have control over. While you play a role in many people's lives, you do not control them and, therefore, are not responsible for what those people do with their own lives.

When you begin taking responsibility for yourself, however, you may also want to take responsibility for things unrelated to you. You may see yourself as responsible for fixing other people's problems because you want to be liked by them. Maybe it is because you want a particular end result and believe that if you want something done right, you need to do it yourself. Or maybe it is because you want to be a good person and help out other people.

Remember what we discussed about how being selfless is selfish? Remember also what we discussed about how helping others to help themselves has a lasting effect on their lives? Well, give other people the chance to grow by giving them the opportunity to take responsibility for their own lives. Exhibit your support for others through encouragement and assistance. From there, it is up to them to take over because they are in control of their own lives. That is the difference between helping and doing.

The topic of whom you are responsible for naturally lends itself to a conversation about parenting as parents have a responsibility to their children. When it comes to parenting, a parent's responsibility in raising a child exists only so far in that the child is a result of its parents procreating or adopting it. And the responsibility for that action also requires responsibility for the repercussions of that action. A child, however, is another person, meaning even a parent doesn't have control over him/her.

Parents often try to control their children as long as they can, typically until the children begin to develop in adolescence and rebel against such controlling. The truth is that a parent is responsible for raising a child, but a child is still responsible for his/her own actions. In this way, a parent's obligation to his/her child is the same as the concept of helping others to help themselves. Even in raising a child, the child needs to learn to live for him/herself. A parent's job is to teach, encourage, and assist—but not to control.

Regret
Another side effect of taking responsibility for your life is the possibility of regret. You may look back on your actions, blame yourself for what went wrong, and wish you had acted differently. But this only hands control of your life over to your past. When you make a decision, you only have the evidence provided to you at the time. And right now, your responsibility is in what you do with what is presented to you in this moment.

Regret is simply taking responsibility for the action but not for the correction. It is blaming yourself and not doing anything about what has happened. It's missing half of the responsibility opportunity. Responsibility doesn't just precede a situation in terms of preparation; it also follows the situation in terms of response.

You are not just responsible for what you have done. You are responsible for what you do now. That's what makes responsibility so great. It doesn't merely condemn you for mistakes; it reminds you to do something about them and move on.

Mistakes are truly just unfinished projects. You complete them when you are no longer affected by your past. To blame inward or outward is to both fight and cry over what has happened. Responsibility is not simply about laying blame; it's about doling out control over everyone who is affected by what has happened. Give yourself that power, and do something great for yourself and for others.

When you regret, what you fail to realize is that had you taken an alternative path, you would likely regret that choice too because regret doesn't come from having made bad choices; it comes from having a bad perspective. With regret, you look at circumstances and focus on the negativity you believe is causing you pain rather than focusing on your ability to do something about your pain.

Forgiveness

There are three types of situations that make you feel bad: 1.) When you have caused someone else to feel bad, 2.) When someone or something has caused you to feel bad, and 3.) When you have caused yourself to feel bad. In all these scenarios, "you" play a role; and it is up to you to get past the situation's drain on your life.

When you can find your role in causing the problems that affect you, it is up to you to correct the situation. However, there is not always much you can do to improve negative situations other than to apologize. Sometimes that's your best means of taking responsibility. Saying you're sorry can often give you control over situations that seem out of control by calming everyone down. Sometimes you owe an apology to others, and sometimes you owe an apology to yourself. However, once you admit your errors and ask forgiveness, you must always grant yourself that forgiveness.

As I mentioned in the last chapter, you must make amends with yourself to be able to let go of your past. Responsibility is what gives you control of situations, but forgiveness is what allows you to move on from them. By forgiving yourself for your mistakes, you admit that you're not perfect and accept yourself as you are. Giving yourself credit for your effort and relief from your past is what gives you the freedom to enjoy this moment and every moment that follows it.

The longer you wait to forgive yourself, the longer the wait will be until you are free to stop focusing on the negative events that have transpired in your life. But let's be honest; most of us don't want to forgive ourselves until we feel okay with everything that has happened. Unfortunately, that type of progression is much slower than doing the opposite. Forgiving yourself *first* is the fast route to happiness.

The Chapter Break early in this book had a paragraph, which I told you to read out loud. It was about forgiving yourself. It's something we all need to do in life because taking responsibility for your own life means doing your best to improve it. And when you leave the negativity of the past behind you, you're doing what's best for you. But there is no technique to learn how to forgive yourself. It's just something you do, and it begins by saying, "I forgive myself."

While we all encounter troubled times now and then, none of us are truly victims of a negative world; we just don't always realize how much opportunity we have in our lives. Too often we rush to pass off responsibility to avoid being the reason we feel bad; we ignore responsibility because we don't want to make an effort, and we deny responsibility to displace our fears of failure. We sit around and wait for others to take responsibility instead, yet our feelings are no one's responsibility but our own.

It's time to stop depending on others and start "independing." Be the one to take charge of your life by taking responsibility for it. Embrace the role you have in every situation. The decisions you make come from within you. The actions you take come from within you. And when you can acknowledge how much responsibility you have for your experiences, you realize how much control you really have in what you decide, what you do, and how you feel. Responsibility means embracing the fact that you have created your life and that you decide what you do with it from here.

Responsibility is the greatest gift that is most given up in this world.

Chapter 21

There's Freedom in Failure

Everything you do in this world comes from your own effort. It's what makes you who you are. And when you put forth that effort, it is always in the pursuit of some opportunity. Many times, however, we don't see opportunity. We see loneliness; we see disappointment, and we see loss. We see this negativity when we see ourselves as incapable of success. We associate our own failure with negativity. And when we see failure as part of our character, we don't view that negativity as simply a momentary experience; we fear it will carry on for the rest of our lives. It is this fear that removes all possibility from our sights, thereby blinding us from opportunity. And without opportunity in view, what reason is there to put forth effort?

Energy is your currency in life, and effort is the use of that energy. But putting forth effort doesn't mean having a good life; it means living well. So take a moment right now and ask yourself if you are happy with the way you live? Don't ask yourself whether you are happy with your life. That's a perspective that focuses on past results. Your real opportunity for appreciation lies in what you do with your life now. So in this moment, ask yourself that question: "Am I happy with the way I live?"

Your Effort

We put forth effort in this world to make our dreams a reality. We do it to achieve our goals. Whether the desire is to become popular, rich, or just plain happy, we put forth effort not to fail but to succeed.

But sometimes we do fail. What come of our actions are tools to learn more about ourselves, this world, and how we interact. Life, however, does not end after success or failure. Success and failure are results, and therefore, they are only as valuable as what you do with them.

While success and failure are what so many people use to judge themselves and the world around them, those results are not definitive. Those results only last until you begin living again, until you begin doing something new with your time. You are only tied to past results if you spend your time looking back instead of making the most of what exists in this moment. The past says nothing more than what was. A future experience will likewise not define you. What are failure and success really but when you give up trying?

Accepting the inevitability of change in this world means accepting failure as a possibility. Just as we discussed that considering the possibilities of what might happen in life is what allows you to be open to change, accepting the possibility of failure is what protects you against the pain of failure when it happens.

You might question why you would want to be okay with failure, believing it would take the value out of succeeding. It doesn't. The reason you put forth effort is to succeed, but realizing that failure is not the end of the world is what allows you to pick yourself up and try again if you fail.

In life, you will make mistakes. You will lose what you have. You will do your best, and people will still complain. No matter what you do, how hard you try, or how good your intention, now and again you will fall flat on your face. And you need to know that when that happens, it's really not that bad.

Your Failure

Failure comes in many forms. It can feel like loss, rejection, weakness, stupidity, incompetence, or just plain not getting your way. And for many, when they strive for success and fail, they lose all faith in themselves to persevere beyond that failure. They blame themselves, fearing that their failure is the unavoidable result of who they are. They characterize themselves not by their effort but by their experience.

Some may instead blame others for their failure. In an attempt to alleviate their own accountability, they look for a scapegoat. They see other people as the cause of their own failure, making themselves victims because they believe it is better to have failed because of someone else's doing than to be responsible for their lives not being the way they want.

But whether you see yourself as a failure or a victim, both are a matter of perspective and neither is a fair characterization of who you are. You see, failure is a part of life. It's inevitable. Once you accept this fact, failure no longer weighs on you as much. Accepting that you will fail in life means being okay with failing, and that gives you the power to determine if failure is the end of your experience or merely a hurdle for you to overcome.

When many of us lose friends, lovers, jobs, and what's important to us, we often sulk and sometimes fall into depression. It paralyzes us from moving forward. But what if you already knew ahead of that loss that failure to maintain its existence in your life would be okay? What if you knew that you could survive anything, even losing everything? I mean, hey, you have suffered through depression and made it this far. If you thought this way, when the time came that you lost what you had, the blow might still be hard to bear; but it wouldn't be life-shattering. When you experience loss and it's not so bad, you give it another shot. You don't have to give up when you lose. You can try again and again and again.

In the 20th century, the New York Yankees won more World Series championships than any other team in baseball; but they also lost more World Series championships than any other team.[1] It was their effort that got them to the World Series in the first place. The fact is that trying means occasionally failing, but if you never try, you'll never succeed. No matter how many setbacks you have, only your effort can carry you through to a life you appreciate; and that's really what makes your life a success.

People often give failure so much meaning because they see it as a result that determines something about their lives. They fear its significance and would rather walk away than try and fail. But in either case, they would be failing: failure by trying or failure by not trying. In life, it will be both your effort and acceptance of failure that allow you to do anything without anything else getting in your way. There is a world of possibility around you and by taking your focus off the significance of loss, you can clearly see those opportunities before you.

Think about all those rags-to-riches stories you hear about. They occur not merely because people are trying to pull themselves out of poverty; these stories exist because those people have already experienced failure. They lived with failure and learned to accept it. They put forth the effort to become rich and succeeded because they knew that if they failed, nothing would change. They would be okay. There was nothing to lose and, therefore, only one direction to go.

Now you might think that you have plenty to lose, but what do you really have that you value and is truly irreplaceable? Think about your list of priorities when you contemplate this question. Once you determine your answer, don't replace those things and don't risk them either. But when it comes to everything else (the places you live, the possessions you own, the plans you have), don't let those things get in the way of you pushing yourself. If you do, you will be gripped by fear that by doing anything in life, you risk losing what you have.

When you feel as though your life will not be okay if you lose what you have, failure is tied directly to your self-esteem. If being unsuccessful is inevitable at some point in your life, holding the belief that failure is not okay means you are destined to be depressed. In fact, if you define yourself by what you do and you see failure as a negative commentary on what you are doing with your life, failure does not just feel like failing at an endeavor; it feels like failing as a human being.

When you accept the inevitability of failure, however, you keep moving forward. You refuse to embrace excuses as a means to rationalize your failure. Taking responsibility is about taking back control of your life from others. Accepting failure is about taking back control of your life from your fears. What matters is not failure but how you let failure affect your next steps. Failure is not an indication of what you are; it's just what happens.

Failure is a good thing because it means you're not perfect. You are aloud to make mistakes. You don't need to succeed, and you won't always succeed. You are aloud to be wrong, and it's okay to fail. You don't have to be anyone other than who you are. You don't need to do anything anyone says you should be doing. And you don't have to be great at what you do.

Having the freedom to screw up allows you to push the limits of possibility. You work harder knowing that failure isn't so bad whereas when you fear failure, you rarely try that hard. When you fear failure, you tend to give up easily or quit after achieving only moderate success, believing that some success is better than putting forth lots of energy and losing. The interesting thing, however, is that fearing failure can sometimes cause you to make less of an effort than you believe you're actually making.

When I think about this concept, I am reminded of the first time I did a headstand. While the general idea of doing a headstand may seem silly, the lesson I derived from it was significant on my view of life. I vividly remember that moment as I placed my head and my hands on the ground and kicked my legs up into the air. I was careful not to kick too high because I didn't want to go toppling over onto my back. But I tried and tried, unable to balance my legs above my body. Each time I went to kick my legs up, they quickly came back down to the ground.

Then I decided to kick my legs up into the air as high as I could, accepting that I might kick too hard and flip over. So I cleared everything out of the way to prepare for failure so that if I did topple over onto my back, I didn't hurt myself too badly. And then I kicked my legs up high into the air. And you know what? That was the moment I did my first headstand.

There are two perspectives in this story: how high I thought I was kicking and how high I was actually kicking. All that time that I had initially been trying to do a headstand, I wasn't kicking my legs up nearly high enough. Someone watching me easily could have seen the problem, but from my point of view, I thought it was just my inability to do a headstand. I thought my fear of not kicking my legs up higher was rational to keep me safe, but it was that fear that was keeping me from doing what I was trying to do. It was my acceptance of the possibility of failure and my preparation for how I would handle it that allowed me to succeed.

Fear is not bad; it helps set boundaries to protect you from getting hurt, but if you always succumb to fear, you'll never get anywhere either. Sometimes in life, we all need to take chances. Look at your surroundings and your strengths, and you'll begin to see how significant the risks of failure are versus the feeling of having not tried. Sometimes you will get hurt, but your willingness to accept failure is what will allow you to dust yourself off and move on. If you never take any risks in life, you'll never move. If you never push yourself, you'll never move forward. Now is the time to make your move.

Embracing failure does not mean trying to fail, nor is it knowing that you will fail at any specific goal; it is simply being okay with the possibility of failing. If you knew for sure that you would fail, you wouldn't try; and many people live their lives this way. They think they aren't good enough the way they are and see failure as imminent. Now the fact that they see failure in their future is a good thing, but they are viewing failure wrong. They see it as inevitable and, therefore, a reason not to try rather seeing failure's inevitability as providing the freedom to fail, allowing them to try as many times as they like. One perspective focuses on result and one sees effort. One perspective is paralyzing and the other is freeing.

When you give up the fear of failure, you consequently give up the fear in trying. You can pursue your dreams further than you might have otherwise, knowing that if you fail after effort, it means nothing about who you are. Failure can be a breeding ground for depression or an inconsequential result. You decide what it is for you.

When It's Okay to Give Up and When It's Not

While failure doesn't mean you have to give up, it's also okay to give up. Being okay with failure means recognizing this. Some people dedicate themselves to an idea and refuse to give up because they are unwilling to fail. They stay in situations they hate because of the fear of what might happen if they walked away. They believe that any effort they already put forth would be in vain if they gave up, but effort is what makes giving up okay. It is the effort that has been made that provides you with the knowledge of what is good for you and what isn't, what you want and what you don't want, and what is worth more effort and what is not.

Eventually and particularly with negative patterns, it's best to throw in the towel, accept failure, and move on. That's how you have new experiences. Otherwise, you spend your life feeling miserable, trying to create a future that just isn't going to happen. Every now and then, you might look back and wonder what would have happened had you remained committed to something; but if you are unhappy, embracing failure will bring you relief and open you up to new paths that can offer happiness.

Commitment is all part of truly making an effort, but if your effort is sustained purely because of the fear of what failure would mean for your life, you have missed the point of effort. Effort is what makes you who you are whereas the freedom to fail allows you to discover who you are by putting that effort toward any path you choose.

Sometimes, even before you make an effort, opportunities are presented that you just aren't interested in pursuing. That's okay too. Not everything is worth putting forth all your energy. It's okay to say "no." There are always other options in this world. You get to determine what is best for you, but there is a big difference between giving up because you are satisfied and giving up because you are afraid of losing what you have.

For years I struggled with the concept of when you are letting go of something that's not meant to be and when you are giving up too easily. I looked for the subtle differences, trying to find that fine line that distinguished the two until one day I realized that letting go and giving up are the same thing. What makes them appear different is whether you view walking away from something as an opportunity or a loss. The action, however, is the same. The perspective that makes failure an opportunity comes directly from the knowledge that your life will be okay even if you don't get what you want.

So how do you get to the point of being able to accept failure in your life? Well, you already made a list of how bad events in your life led to good experiences. You read a whole chapter on accepting change. The chapters on hope and doubt focused on helping you reduce the meaning you put into what you accomplish or don't accomplish by focusing on what you are doing in the present. It's all related because your life follows a path. Either you try or you don't try. And either you disregard the significance of failure or you magnify it.

Your Success
The ability to overcome the fear of failure will play an important role in your happiness, but equally important will be your ability to overcome the need for success. Just as easily as failure can stop you from trying by convincing you that you can't succeed, success can cause you to stop trying by convincing you that there is nothing more to do. Achieving your goals can lead to complacency in life because you think you are on top. You plateau and stop putting forth effort. And then who are you if you're not doing anything?

Success is less about believing it represents you; it's about wanting it to represent you. We all want to prove to ourselves and to the world that we are capable of accomplishing whatever we set out to do. But beyond the initial moment of success, what you accomplish will not affect how you feel about yourself; it will be your effort to maintain success if you succeed that displays true self-pride. For many, however, this can make success feel like a burden. Once they succeed, they then place pressure on themselves to remain successful. And so they end up both fearing failure *and* lamenting success.

Does this mean that it's best never to succeed? Of course not. The problem with success, much like with failure, is simply the emphasis we all tend to put on it. Giving yourself credit for your accomplishments is important, but giving yourself credit for your effort is more important. You will win and lose in this life, and whatever the outcome, all that matters is that you don't give up on yourself. That's how you take the next step of your life, learning to appreciate yourself for who you are, not just what you've done.

While there will always be some people waiting out there on the sidelines ready to point out what they believe represents you, what truly matters is what you think of yourself. And when you look at your life, can you say that you are happy with the way you live? That's what matters. You're what matters because you are, in fact, whatever you do.

Your life is about giving and taking, doing and appreciating, holding on to what matters and letting go of what doesn't. When you give up the need to succeed, you succeed just by being who you are. You acknowledge yourself by how you are spending your time, and that is something you have full control over.

You won't always get what you seek in this world, but being okay with that means being okay with life, which makes living so much easier. It will be your effort toward succeeding and acceptance of failure that will carry you from a life of unease to one that flows. In fact, every concept in this book is guided by the willingness to do your best and being okay with whatever happens. Your effort to learn about yourself and this world and accept whatever you find, your effort to overcome obstacles and accept your role in unwanted circumstances, your effort to prepare for possible change and accept change that has taken place, and your effort to honor your principles and accept that you won't always get your way are all part of the same path that lays your depression to rest and gives you back that smile you lost.

Free yourself from the demand of success. Give up the fear of failure. The need to be perfect is stressful. It breeds doubt, fear, and depression. Breathe easy, do your best, and know that you, and only you, decide whether failure is the end of your effort.

Everything you need to succeed in this world is in you. There is always room to grow, and that gives you reason to put forth effort. You have the freedom to fail, and that gives you the freedom to do your best. The ability to overcome your fears, your challenges, and your depression comes down to an enthusiastic amount of effort and this simple understanding of failure. Gaze upon this world now and from this point forward and see what has been blinded from so much of your life: opportunity.

*The key to happiness is doing your best
without needing to be the best.*

Chapter 22

The Return of Depression

For me, this book started off as a project in which I was keeping notes on the lessons I learned from my experiences in an effort to avoid making the same mistakes again. But during the times when I needed to review those notes most, I ignored their existence, going about life how I pleased with disastrous results. I occasionally wrote in a journal but failed to ever read it. What I remembered from my past made new experiences easier to handle than past ones, but it wasn't enough. When I finally looked back on those notes and read through my journal, it was amazing to find that I had literally written down exactly what would happen were I to take certain paths or avoid others. It was my memory that could not keep up with the lessons of my past experiences. The truth is that you can have all the answers in the world, but unless you are willing to live by them, your life won't ever be what you know it can be.

I spent nearly all my life critical of others, harsh on myself, untrusting, wishing for what I lost or gave up, and ignoring so much of what the world was offering me. And to this day, I remember sitting on my bed, accepting a hug from a friend, and whispering under my breath over and over, "I don't want to do this to myself anymore."

The path that you and I have taken together has been because of your doing. It has been your effort that brought you to the end of this book. It has been your commitment that helped you to learn about your relationship with the world around you. It has been your genuineness that enabled you to face yourself, learn about yourself, and appreciate everything that you are. And this is all something to be proud of. It's okay to smile about this.

The path, however, does not end when this book ends. It continues as long as you continue to learn and apply that knowledge to your life. You've undoubtedly gained a great deal of insight from reading this book, writing in your journal, and answering questions you've asked of yourself. You've worked hard for this knowledge, and you probably won't remember most of it in a month.

You see, we need reasons to do things in life. And when you start feeling better about yourself, you lose that reason that initially propelled you to strive for a better life. So it becomes easy to ignore the work that needs to continue being done. You stop keeping your journal, you stop taking care of your body, and you leave things like your Yes/No "After the Fact" lists at home. You may have already given up some of the techniques you began using early on in this book. You may have already forgotten many of the concepts you learned in the first few chapters. It's a lot; I know this, but it's all connected.

You began walking this path because you were tired of feeling bad and wanted to change your life. But change can go both ways. Consider that living well mentally is similar to living well physically. If you are overweight and go on a diet, you will probably lose weight; but if you revert to your old eating habits, you will likely return to your original weight. Similarly with depression, if you don't continue the work of living well, it will come back.

This may not be what you want to hear, but it's the truth. Depression is not something that goes away. It is replaced by living well, which means that depression has the ability to return if you disregard the work you've done and the knowledge you've gained. If you go back to living the way you did in the past, you'll start having those familiar feelings of depression creeping back into your life.

You'll lay your head down in the middle of the day just wanting to get away from everything. You'll start contemplating doing unhealthy things, disregarding your own well-being and that of others. You'll feel lonely, sad, mad, and uneasy at random times; and you will know these are signs of depression on the horizon. These familiar feelings of depression are warnings that you have gone astray with your principles, priorities, and patterns. And if you don't pay attention to these warnings, depression can set in fast. You'll have to sit up, consider what thoughts or actions might have led to your feelings, and make the necessary changes to feel better; you've worked too hard to get over this.

For many people, however, once they start overcoming depression, they stop recognizing their role in how they feel. They fail to correlate their actions with their feelings and end up believing that no matter what they do, they are destined to be depressed. Naturally, they then stop trying to do anything to improve their lives; and that's when depression really sets in.

I promise that you are in no way destined to be depressed. But your life comes from what you do with it, and when you don't take care of yourself, you get sick with depression. You cannot rely on a past that is good or bad to determine who you are now. It's what you do in this moment that determines whether you are living well. You know all this, and it's up to you to apply it to your life. You can do this. You wouldn't have gotten through this book otherwise. But you need to believe it. So go on, tell yourself that you believe in yourself.

There will be times in your life when you feel utterly alone. There will also be times when you feel loved and surrounded by friends. *Both* of these experiences are important for your journey through life. They are opportunities to learn about yourself and yourself in relation to others in a constantly changing world. They are the two ways you grow.

When you feel bad, it is the most crucial time to take a step back and think about what you were just doing that might have contributed to your feeling of uneasiness. What were you thinking about? Whom were you speaking with?

Take time away from some of your scheduled activities to get outside and read over your journal and through this book. Take the time to reflect on your life. Consider what you have been doing with your time that might be contrary to the steps you took toward bettering yourself.

When you encounter any obstacle in life, there will always be a reason for your predicament. But you are not bound to what exists in the past and you are not bound to what may come in the future. All you are bound to is who you are in this moment and what you do with the time you have.

The more you are able to remember and follow through on actions that exhibit living well, the more you will be happy with the person you are and the life you live. The process is easier said than done, however, because it is lifelong. You will continuously have to make decisions that honor your principles, look for opportunities in changes you didn't anticipate, take the time to recognize what is important, and consider which paths are bringing you growth and happiness and which are preventing you from that.

This book is not meant to tell you how to live. That is your choice. This book is a guide to help you take control of your life. And so I encourage you to hold on to this copy for yourself. As you turn back to it throughout your life, you are likely to find that many of the concepts make more sense; and you will also likely see many of those concepts taking shape in your life.

Your journey is not on the pages in this book though. You know this, and I know this. There is no substitute for the intensity of life's experiences, but it doesn't mean you have to walk this path blindly. The words in this book and those in your journal will hold more permanency than your reactionary mood to the circumstances you face. Living well is not always easy, but it creates a life that feels strong in activities and wonderful in silence.

Destruction happens quickly.
Creation takes time, effort, and patience.

Chapter 23

Moving On and Finding Freedom

Experiencing depression isn't anything anyone ever plans for. It's not a choice anyone would make for themselves, but it's what came into our lives. And sometimes that's just the way it is; life throws you a curveball, and you don't have a clue what to do. It's when you want to walk away most, but it's also when you need yourself most.

Whatever you encounter, it is up to you to get yourself through this life. Letting go of depression requires that you look within yourself and understand what your emotions are signifying. It means looking around, accepting what has happened, and determining how to make the most of your circumstances. Depression allows you to see that when you lose everything, all you have is yourself. And in the one moment that exists, you decide what you do with yourself.

There are no rules in life. Those things you never contemplated to be possible can happen before your very eyes. And while anything is possible, you won't always get the life you seek. You might actually get something better, which you didn't know existed. Whatever is to come, you will never know exactly what will happen throughout the rest of your life. There may not even be a rest of your life. But in every moment, you have a choice. That choice is simply what to do. And while so many of us search for reasons to make a specific choice, the details are all secondary to the simple choice of who you choose to be.

Change will bring about fluctuations in your mood, your health, and every relationship you have. But before you react to all the frustrations, challenges, and opportunities you encounter, you must accept that all three of these experiences are the same. A conflict can appear as a frustration you have to deal with, a challenge to get your message across, or an opportunity for growth. What makes them appear different is how you view them. What determines their effect on your life is how you react to them. And just as your feelings affect your actions, so too do your actions affect your feelings.

On the path from depression to living well, you will experience several emotions; but your obligation to yourself has always been about being genuine. When you first confronted yourself, you may have met someone sad, scared, and lonely. But as you worked on yourself, that person began changing. And as you make your way out of depression, you begin to meet someone new. You act and think differently, sometimes without conscious effort. And while you may appreciate your new self, you also may encounter an overwhelming sense of fear at who you have become. You may not recognize this new person and fear that you've lost yourself. But I assure you, that's just the feeling of growth.

As debilitating as depression can be, over time it becomes familiar. You have spent much of your life doing things without reason, looking back at what you did wrong, and wavering in your opportunities about what to do next. But when you act based on your principles rather than purely on your circumstances, that instability becomes your past.

The fear of having lost who you were in exchange for a new way of living is all part of taking the next step in your life. That fear is real. It's genuine. It's a sign that what you are doing is important. And while the difference between depression and discomfort may initially feel slight, when you focus on how your actions make you feel and not just the change in lifestyle, you can clearly see which direction you're facing. When you pay less attention to your comfort and more attention to your principles, you exude confidence in this transformed you. And confidence is the one place fear cannot exist.

Freedom

Being, knowing, and accepting yourself are the foundations of a good life. Using these foundations, you gain the opportunity to control your life rather than living at the whim of this world. Just like the need to get something for giving, when you cross the boundary of fear, you give up depression and gain freedom. Living well gives you the freedom to reclaim your life as your own, a life that you can create as you see fit and be proud of the way you live it.

Freedom, however, comes with one great opportunity and one great responsibility. The opportunity is choice. You have the opportunity to do whatever you want in this world. While some of the choices you make will have a profound effect on your life, remember not to put so much emphasis on choice that it overwhelms you. The significance you give to what your choices might lead to down the road will only make you doubt and fear what you do and don't do. Just embrace the actualization of your principles and your life will flow from the great opportunity of freedom: the choice of who you want to be.

The one responsibility that comes with freedom is accepting other people's personal freedom. You must accept that their views and choices may not coincide with yours. They may disagree with you or you may disagree with how they choose to live their lives. Still, you must accept that not everyone is where you are emotionally, not everyone will ever be where you are, and many people do not believe that where you are is where one should be. But the way you view this world is not for them to decide. Nor is it for you to decide how they should feel or what they should believe.

You hear all the time how people fight and die for freedom, but too many people give it up because of what it means. Freedom means that everyone gets to be whomever they choose to be. Most people want to control others, judge others, and believe that their freedom is compromised by the freedom of others. But when people do this, they inadvertently give up their own freedom.

Letting go of depression really means letting go. You let go of the way you thought life should have been. You let go of the significance of the past, the future, or anything that doesn't exist. You let go of the belief that what you have should make you who you are.

Your life is your own to do with it what you will. There is no pressure other than the pressure you put on yourself. There is no hate other than the hate you use to avoid looking within. There is no doubt other than the doubt you cast over a significance that may not actually exist. There is no moment other than the moment in which you are living.

This world has so much mystery in it, so many things we will never understand. But what we can understand can only come from exploring, questioning, and being open to what we never expected to happen bringing us everything we never knew we wanted. It's up to you to pull through and do what you believe in this moment is right for you. This world will change just as your feelings will change, and you can't worry about what's not yet here or what's already gone. All you can do is the best with what you have. That's not something you judge; that's something you believe in.

You will learn so much about life outside this book. I, like you, am just trying to figure out the journey as I go along. Your effort that you put in every day to explore, accept, and interact with whatever you encounter is what allows you to peacefully coexist with this world. It's what allows you to say "no" to the paths that lead to depression. It's what allows you to say "yes" to yourself. It's what allows you to relax and to smile.

That person you were—the one you almost gave up on—has been strengthened. You breathed life back into the person you were and are creating the person you are. You made a commitment to yourself when you began this book, and you kept it. And because of your commitment, the relationship you have with yourself has developed into something you can appreciate as you become someone you appreciate.

This book may end, but your life continues; and that means the work is constant. The end of this book, like everything in life, is simply a step in your journey. And outside these pages is a world waiting for you to step up and be the person you envision yourself being. The world won't always give you everything you want though; *you* have to make the effort. But if you focus on your effort to pursue not just what you want from this world but the type of person you want to be, the world won't need to give you anything. You will already have all the tools you need.

You are in the driver's seat of this moment. You decide who you are and you express that decision in everything you do. You can be anyone you want to be, lead any life you choose. This is the path of overcoming depression, but it is also the journey of developing your relationships with yourself and with everything around you. It is a journey that you are writing every day in your journal, in your mind, and in your heart. It's here and it's real and it's now. It's the journey we call life.

It's not always like this, but it is now.

Notes

Throughout my writing of this book, I kept notes about the experience and wanted to share a few of those notes with you. It was quite fascinating to me how many of the concepts I was writing about also served as lessons to help me through the process of writing this book. But like I said in Chapter 1, "this book is not so much about me as it is about life." Enjoy.

***

Upon telling someone once that I was writing a book on overcoming depression, I was asked whether I had been through depression. And I said, "Yes." That person then asked me, "And you overcame it?" And I said, "I will have overcome it when I finish the book because I can't finish the book until I do."

***

While I had a significant background of knowledge that I had gained from my own life experiences, I did not start this book with all the answers. In fact, I don't expect to ever have all the answers. This book developed as I wrote it because of my effort to continue learning about life each day. And truthfully, this book was often encouragement for me to learn about the way we interact with ourselves and our surroundings.

***

I made the choice not to look into how or with whom to get this book published until I was done writing it because I didn't want to think too big and end up doubting myself. I set out to write a book to help both myself and others. And published or not, that was my goal.

***

I needed to be okay with this book not being perfect. It was the only way to move on.

***

I experienced doubt about finishing the chapter on doubt. And I knew that if I could finish that chapter, I would have written it correctly because I would have solved what I was trying to explain how to solve.

***

The end of Chapter 20 references the word "independing." This is a word I created on Groundhog Day 2010. It is the action form of the word independent. I find it interesting that there is no verb form of the word "independent" in dictionaries and fully support the inclusion of such a word.

Much of this book is about effort, and I don't believe that it is enough to simply depend on ourselves. I believe it is essential that we look at ourselves not as reliant but as capable. It's time that each of us took responsibility for our own lives and took pride in that.

So let's formally bring together "Me," "Myself," and "I" and all that they do. Let's get together once and for all and independ. It even has a catchy ring to it, sure to be the next new dance craze. It'll just be people dancing with themselves.

So Dear: Merriam-Webster, How do you do: Oxford, Good Evening: Mr. and Mrs. Wikipedia, let's officially make "independing" a word.

Independing: (intr.v) To depend on oneself: I'm independing to get through this difficult task; or, I independ to get myself to work every day.

***

"Lenting," first appearing in Chapter 5, is another word I created. I modified the word Lent into a verb because, similar to *independing*, it is the effort we must make that matters. To me, the holiday of Lent is not as important as the knowledge that giving up something from your life creates for you (at least in the context of this book). In a world in which what you do makes you who you are, lenting is a very real action that can have a profound effect on the way you view what you have in your life.

***

I dedicated so much of my time and energy to writing this book that I was forced to cut short my time doing other activities. I gave up parties, vacations, hobbies, intimate relationships, and quality time with my friends and family. It was something I didn't want to do, but I made the choice that what was best for me was to focus on this book.

Now you may recall me saying in this book that one of the biggest advances I made in overcoming my depression was when I stopped putting so much emphasis on what people thought of me. Well, the technique of "lenting" in the fifth chapter is about taking space from your normal activities to evaluate the importance of what you have in your life. This was a big part of what I was doing with my life by writing this book. I was lenting. I was giving up so much of what I wanted to be doing, and that allowed me to appreciate the people in my life without putting so much emphasis on them that I feared their judgments.

Through this journey that I took, I became my best friend—someone I could always count on—and I believe *that* will help to improve my relationships with everyone and everything else.

***

This has been one of the most challenging, time-consuming, and greatest experiences of my life.

***

One evening a long time ago, about a year before I started writing this book, I was up late doing some deep thinking when I came to what I believed was the key to happiness. Broken down as simply as possible, I saw it as "doing your best without expectation." The next day, I went out and bought a key to wear around my neck to remind myself of this. Every time someone would ask me what the key was to, I would tell them and simultaneously remind myself of the key to happiness.

I wore that key around my neck every day of my life for the next two years until I gave it away. Without the key to remind me of how to be happy, I continued to study life, open to whatever I found. But what I discovered was that in every frustration, challenge, and opportunity, what allowed me to get to the next step with appreciation for my life was putting forth my own effort and accepting whatever happened. It seemed that the expectation I needed to give up was the need for perfection. And so I realized that the true key to happiness is *doing your best without needing to be the best.*

I wore this concept within me every day after that until one day I looked across my room and saw a plaque sitting on my dresser. This plaque had been handed down from my grandfather to my father to me, and on it were written the words of the Serenity Prayer. That's when I noticed that those words were the key to happiness as well, only said differently.

> *"God grant me the serenity to accept the things I*
> *cannot change, courage to change the things I can,*
> *and wisdom to know the difference."*
> > *–attributed to Reinhold Niebuhr*[1]

I had this prayer sitting in my room as far back as I can remember, but it did no good. I wore a key around my neck for years, but it did no good. And now I have a book that I have written, and it likewise will do no good unless I internalize and exhibit everything I now know. Like I said in Chapter 22, "you can have all the answers in the world, but unless you are willing to live by them, your life won't ever be what you know it can be." It is the effort you make in this life that makes you who you are, but only when you accept yourself and this world do you realize how true that is.

***

As I drew near the completion of this book, I found myself frustrated, seemingly unable to finish. I felt a sense of separation anxiety looming from having worked on it nearly every day for more than three and a half years. I also had the draw of new projects in sight as I longed to finish this book so that I could move on to them. Pulled in two directions, I was stuck.

What helped bring me through this rough patch was reminding myself that I set out to *write* a book, not to *finish* a book. Of course, finishing was important; but the finished product was a result—and this life is about effort. I was the one who determined when the book was finished, and if I wanted to be done, the simplest and most direct way to do that was to just say, "I'm done." But I didn't. I pushed through by not focusing on the future but the moment that I was in, that moment when I was writing this book.

***

I set so many deadlines for myself to finish this book, and I missed every one of them. I worked so hard some days as they passed into nights until the sun began to rise outside my window while my eyes squinted, staring blankly at a computer screen. Learning about life takes time, and sometimes I just didn't have the answers I needed. But with each personal deadline that came and went, I kept putting forth effort, believing that the next deadline was the one. But you can't rush life. And besides, going after the goal with so much effort and being okay with not reaching that milestone I set for myself was what this was all about. My acceptance and my effort together is what allowed me to write the words: *The End*...which, of course, is just another step.

***

The End

For more information about Josh Blumenthal, visit
www.JoshBlumenthal.com

References

CHAPTER 1: WHY CAN'T I JUST BE HAPPY?

[1] Antidepressants: What you need to know about depression medications. (n.d.). *Helpguide.org: A trusted non-profit resource*. Retrieved November 22, 2010, from http://helpguide.org/mental/medications_depression.htm

CHAPTER 2: PHYSICALLY INDUCED MOTIVATION

[1] Jegtvig, S. (2007, March 15). Drinking water to maintain good health. *Nutrition—About nutrition and diet*. Retrieved June 11, 2010, from http://nutrition.about.com /od/hydrationwater/a/waterarticle.htm

[2] Reynolds, G. (2004). All about hydration. *Life Time Fitness—Feel good inside*. Retrieved November 27, 2010, from http://www.lifetimefitness.com/magazine/index.cfm?strWe bAction=article_detail&intArticleId=254

[3] Water can heal: Water and depression, stress and anxiety. (n.d.). *Freedrinkingwater.com*. Retrieved November 14, 2008, from http://www.freedrinkingwater.com/water-education3/21-water-and-depression-stress-anxiety.htm

[4] Water: How much should you drink every day?. (n.d.). *Mayo Clinic—Medical information and tools for healthy living*. Retrieved June 11, 2010, from http://www.mayoclinic.com/health/water/NU00283

[5] Burn fat, build lean muscle, and regain your lost energy!. (n.d.). *Weight loss guides and products reviews*. Retrieved

November 29, 2010, from
http://www.weightlossguidesreviews.com/article7.html

6 Moritz, A. (2007). Simple guidelines to avoid gallstones. *The liver and gallbladder miracle cleanse: An all-natural, at-home flush to purify & rejuvenate your body* (p. 142). Berkeley, CA: Ulysses Press.

7 10 reasons to drink water. (n.d.). *All about water—Read, learn, and know about water.* Retrieved November 29, 2010, from http://www.allaboutwater.org/drink-water.html

8 Sahelian, R. (n.d.). Increase dopamine with natural supplements. *Ray Sahelian, M.D., Nutrition expert and best selling author.* Retrieved October 30, 2008, from http://www.raysahelian.com/dopamine.html

9 Dopamine—The 'good feelings' neurotransmitter. (n.d.). *PSPInformation.* Retrieved October 30, 2008, from http://www.pspinformation.com/medications/medications-other/dopamine.shtml

10 Holford, P. (2000). The myth of the well-balanced diet. *The optimum nutrition bible* (p. 31). Freedom, CA: Crossing Press.

11 Vitamin B complex. (n.d.). *Vitamins & health supplements guide.* Retrieved November 22, 2010, from http://www.vitamins-supplements.org/vitamin-B.php

12 Holford, P. (2000). The vitamin scandal. *The optimum nutrition bible* (p. 60). Freedom, CA: Crossing Press.

13 Kurtzweil, P. (1993, May). 'Daily values' encourage healthy diet - Food labels - Includes related information - Focus on food labeling - Cover story. *Find articles at BNET.* Retrieved September 14, 2010, from http://findarticles.com/p/articles/mi_m1370/is_n4_v27/ai_13708934/

14 Holford, P. (2000). Increasing your energy and resistance to stress?. *The optimum nutrition bible* (p. 159). Freedom, CA: Crossing Press.

15 Obikoya, G. (n.d.). Water soluble vitamins. *The Vitamins & Nutrition Center*. Retrieved November 29, 2010, from www.vitamins-nutrition.org/vitamins/water-soluble-vitamins.html

16 Bee pollen—Health supplement information. (n.d.). *Nutritional Supplements Center*. Retrieved November 22, 2010, from http://www.nutritionalsupplementscenter.com/info/HealthSupplement/beepollen.html

17 Fanton, J. P. (2009, March 18). Rhodiola for anxiety, depression and fatigue. *Healthier Talk—Natural health news & community*. Retrieved November 22, 2010, from http://www.healthiertalk.com/rhodiola-21st-century-0403

18 SSRIs. (n.d.). *Health Library*. Retrieved November 29, 2010, from healthlibrary.epnet.com/GetContent.aspx?token=e04 98803-7f62-4563-8d47-5fe33da65dd4&chunkiid=21620

19 Do you really have healthy digestion?. (n.d.). *Healthy for Life*. Retrieved November 22, 2010, from http://www.hfl direct.com/index.php?main_page=index&cPath=124_135

20 Huber, L. (2007, September 13). 5 nutritious habits of the planet's healthiest countries. *CNN*. Retrieved October 30, 2008, from http://www.cnn.com/2007/HEALTH/diet.fitness /08/31/cl.worldly.advice/?imw=Y

21 The 2000 calorie diet. (n.d.). *Livestrong.com—Health, fitness, lifestyle*. Retrieved November 22, 2010, from http://www.livestrong.com/article/303986-the-2000-calorie-diet/

22 10 best foods for energy. (n.d.). *Healthmad*. Retrieved
   November 22, 2010, from
   http://healthmad.com/nutrition/10-best-foods-for-energy/

23 Dolson, L. (2009, July 8). List of high-protein foods and
   amount of protein in each. *Low carb diets at About.com*.
   Retrieved November 22, 2010, from http://lowcarbdiets.
   about.com/od/whattoeat/a/highproteinfood.htm

24 Energy-boosting foods: These 10 foods will keep your motor
   revving all day and all night. (n.d.). *Find articles at BNET*.
   Retrieved June 11, 2010, from http://findarticles.com/p/
   articles/mi_m1608/is_5_19/ai_100545121/?tag=content;col1

25 Refined sugar—The sweetest poison of all.... (n.d.). *Global
   Healing Center—Natural health & organic living*.
   Retrieved October 30, 2008, from www.globalhealingcenter
   .com/refined-sugar-the-sweetest-poison-of-all.html

26 B complex vitamins. (n.d.). *Healthy Vitamins Rx*. Retrieved
   December 23, 2010, from http://www.healthy-vitamins-
   rx.com/html/b-complex-vitamins.html

27 Overview of carbohydrates. (n.d.). *Carbohydrate Counter*.
   Retrieved November 14, 2008, from http://www.carbohydra
   te-counter.org/about-carbohydrates.php

28 Sugar blues. (n.d.). *Natural Nutrition*. Retrieved September
   23, 2010, from http://www.livrite.com/sugar1.htm

29 Mitra, S. (2010, July 28). Parting pangs: Withdrawal
   symptoms of detox. *Complete Wellbeing*. Retrieved
   November 25, 2010, from
   http://completewellbeing.com/article/parting-pangs/

30 Schimelpfening, N. (n.d.). Dual diagnosis creates double
   trouble for the depressed. *About depression—Information
   and support for depression*. Retrieved October 30, 2008,

from http://depression.about.com/cs/drugsalcohol/a/dual diagnosis.htm

[31] The Substance Abuse and Mental Health Services Administration—Homepage. (n.d.). *The Substance Abuse and Mental Health Services Administration.* Retrieved December 2, 2010, from http://www.samhsa.gov/index.aspx

[32] For younger kids: What's so great about the sun, anyway?. (n.d.). *Solar Energy International—Renewable energy education for a sustainable future.* Retrieved November 30, 2010, from http://www.solarenergy.org/younger-kids

[33] Liu, L. (n.d.). Summer sun for winter blues. *MedicineNet.com—We bring doctors' knowledge to you.* Retrieved October 30, 2008, from www.medicinenet.com/ script/main/art.asp?articlekey=50592

[34] Ulrich, C. (2006). The power of touch: Understanding the body-brain connection. *Massage therapy information.* Retrieved November 30, 2010, from http://www.massagetherapy.com/articles/index.php/article _id/1123/The-Power-of-Touch

[35] Scientists find link between dopamine and obesity. (2001, February 1). *Brookhaven National Laboratory—A passion for discovery.* Retrieved October 30, 2008, from http://www.bnl.gov/bnlweb/pubaf/pr/2001/bnlpr020101.htm

[36] Exercise treatment for depression: Efficacy and dose response. (n.d.). *National Center for Biotechnology Information.* Retrieved October 30, 2008, from http://www.ncbi.nlm.nih.gov/pubmed/15626549

[37] Short sleep increases risk of death and over-long sleep can indicate serious illness. (2010, May 5). *Science Daily: Your source for the latest research news.* Retrieved November 22, 2010, from http://www.sciencedaily.com/releases/2010/05/1 00504095109.htm

38 Oversleeping side effects: Is too much sleep harmful?. (n.d.). *WebMD—Better information. Better health.*. Retrieved December 11, 2008, from http://www.webmd.com/sleep-disorders/guide/physical-side-effects-oversleeping?page=2 http://www.webmd.com/sleep-disorders/guide/physical-side-effects-oversleeping?page=2

39 Patlak, M. (2005). *Your guide to healthy sleep*. Washington, D.C.: U.S. Dept. of Health and Human Services, National Institutes of Health, National Heart, Lung, and Blood Institute.

40 Ankrom, S. (2009, June 8). Abdominal breathing—Proper breathing to reduce anxiety. *Panic disorder*. Retrieved December 30, 2010, from http://panicdisorder.about.com/od/livingwithpd/a/deepbreathing.htm

CHAPTER 3: THE VALUE OF RESULTS

CHAPTER 4: PREDICTING THE FUTURE

1 Santayana, G. (1905). Volume 1. *The life of reason; or, The phases of human progress,* (p. 284). New York: C. Scribner's Sons.

2 Schulz, C. *Peanuts*. Retrieved November 29, 2010, from http://peanuts.wikia.com/wiki/File:1107charlie_brown_lucy_football.jpg

3 Layton, J. (n.d.). Is it true that if you do anything for three weeks it will become a habit?. *Discovery Health*. Retrieved September 23, 2010, from health.howstuffworks.com/mental-health/human-nature/behavior/form-a-habit.htm

CHAPTER 5: THE TRUTH ABOUT BAD FOCUS

[1] Lent. (n.d.). *ReligionFacts: Just the facts on religion.* Retrieved September 21, 2010, from http://www.religionfacts.com/christianity/holidays/lent.htm

CHAPTER BREAK: YOUR OPPORTUNITY TO BE HAPPY

CHAPTER 6: KNOW THYSELF

[1] Marks, W. E. (2001). Chapter seven: Is water myth water truth?. *The holy order of water: Healing the earth's waters and ourselves* (p. 91). Great Barrington, MA: Bell Pond Books.

CHAPTER 7: THE BURDEN OF CHOICE

CHAPTER 8: THE FIGHT WITHIN SELF-ESTEEM

[1] Quote details: Bill Cosby: I don't know the.... (n.d.). *The Quotations Page—Your source for famous quotes.* Retrieved September 19, 2010, from http://www.quotationspage.com/quote/603.html

CHAPTER 9: THE SIGNIFICANCE OF DOUBT

CHAPTER 10: THE FATE OF HOPE

[1] The milkmaid and her pail—An Aesop's fable. (n.d.). *Aesop's fables.* Retrieved November 26, 2010, from http://www.aesops-fables.org.uk/aesop-fable-the-milkmaid-and-her-pail.htm

[2] Maslow's hierarchy of needs. (n.d.). *Educational Psychology Interactive.* Retrieved September 23, 2010, from http://www.edpsycinteractive.org/topics/regsys/maslow.html

CHAPTER 11: THE ONLY CONSTANT IS CHANGE

[1] Climate effects on human evolution. (n.d.). *Human evolution by the Smithsonian Institution's human origins program*. Retrieved December 2, 2010, from http://humanorigins.si.edu/research/climate-research/effects

[2] Survival of the adaptable. (n.d.). *What does it mean to be human?*. Retrieved December 2, 2010, from humanorigins.si.edu/sites/default/files/HO_044_055_CHAP_3.pdf

CHAPTER 12: THE PATH OF EXTREMISM

CHAPTER 13: JUDGE NOT, LEST YE BE JUDGED

[1] Carlin, G., Kurtz, B., Carlin B., Hamza, J. (Producers), & Santos, S. J. (Director). (1984). *George Carlin: On campus* [Motion picture]. USA: Mpi Home Video.

CHAPTER 14: THE WORLD DOESN'T REVOLVE AROUND YOU

CHAPTER 15: THE TWO SIDES OF HELP

[1] Quote details: Chinese proverb: Give a man a.... (n.d.). *The Quotations Page—Your source for famous quotes*. Retrieved June 11, 2010, from http://www.quotationspage.com/quote/2279.html

[2] *Speeches that changed the world* (p. 145). (2007). John F. Kennedy. London: Quercus.

CHAPTER 16: LOVE: THE GATEWAY EMOTION

[1] Roberts, A. & Fisher D. (1944). You always hurt the one you love [Recorded by The Mills Brothers]. Decca.

[2] *The Holy Bible: New international version*. (p. 989). (1984). Acts 20:35. Grand Rapids, MI: Zondervan Publishing House.

[3] Leo Durocher quotes. (n.d.). *Baseball Almanac—The official baseball history site*. Retrieved January 8, 2011, from http://www.baseball-almanac.com/quotes/quoduro.shtml

CHAPTER 17: MANAGING YOUR RELATIONSHIPS

CHAPTER 18: COMMUNICATION

[1] Definition of passive-aggressive. (2004, May 8). *MedicineNet.com—We bring doctors' knowledge to you*. Retrieved December 21, 2010, from www.medterms.com/script/main/art.asp?articlekey=32501

[2] Fear of public speaking statistics. (n.d.). *Speech topics help, advice & ideas*. Retrieved June 11, 2010, from http://www.speech-topics-help.com/fear-of-public-speaking-statistics.html

CHAPTER 19: VACATIONING WITH ANGER

[1] Quote details: Mahatma Gandhi: An eye for an.... (n.d.). *The Quotations Page—Your source for famous quotes*. Retrieved September 19, 2010, from http://www.quotationspage.com/quote/30302.html

[2] What does Medusa look like?. (n.d.). *Historyking.com*. Retrieved December 21, 2010, from http://www.historyking.com/Ancient-Greece/Greek-mythology/greek-goddess/medusa/What-Does-Medusa-Look-Like.html

CHAPTER 20: TAKING RESPONSIBILITY

CHAPTER 21: THERE'S FREEDOM IN FAILURE

[1] New York Yankees team history & encyclopedia—Baseball-Reference.com. (n.d.). *Baseball-Reference.com—Major league baseball statistics and history.* Retrieved September 19, 2010, from http://www.baseball-reference.com/teams/NYY/

CHAPTER 22: THE RETURN OF DEPRESSION

CHAPTER 23: MOVING ON AND FINDING FREEDOM

NOTES

[1] Goodstein, L. (2009, November 27). Serenity prayer skeptic now credits Niebuhr. *The New York Times.* Retrieved December 21, 2010, from http://www.nytimes.com/2009/11/28/us/28prayer.html

www.ingramcontent.com/pod-product-compliance
Lightning Source LLC
Chambersburg PA
CBHW022114080426
42734CB00006B/122